JOHN CRAMMER
BERNARD HEINE

The Use of Drugs in Psychiatry

Third Edition

GASKELL

First published 1978
Second edition 1982
Third edition 1991

ISBN 0 902241 37 0
(ISBN 0 902241 02 8 1st and 2nd edn)

Gaskell is an imprint of the Royal College of Psychiatrists,
17 Belgrave Square, London SW1

Distributed in North America
by American Psychiatric Press, Inc.
ISBN 0 88048 604 X

British Library Cataloguing in Publication Data
Crammer, John
The use of drugs in psychiatry.
1. Psychotropic drugs
I. Heine, Bernard II. Royal College of Psychiatrists
615.788

ISBN 0-902241-37-0

Phototypeset by Dobbie Typesetting Limited, Tavistock, Devon
Printed in Great Britain

Contents

Part III. Drug list

Acknowledgements

About 15 years ago, Dr Brian Barraclough first had the idea of this book, and recruited the two of us to help create it. Together we planned what it should be – a practical pocket book that the beginner could consult in clinic or ward. We wrote our selected topics separately, exchanged typescripts and met on several occasions to debate content and expression, so that each final manuscript truly had three authors. It was Brian Barraclough, above all, who emphasised the need for clarity and simplicity. The result was published in 1978, and a new edition in 1982.

Unfortunately, this time, Dr Barraclough has not been able to take part in the final rewriting and editing, although he was able to help in the earlier stages. We are grateful to him for what he did, and for advice also offered by Drs M. Faulk, J. Grimshaw and C. Nunn. Earlier editions were greatly helped by Dr Eric Taylor, Dr E. H. Reynolds, Dr Michael Best and Professors George Fenton, Malcolm Lader and John Corbett, whom we also thank. We have not necessarily adopted their views. However, any errors, distortion or important omissions are ours alone: we hope, of course, that there are none of substance.

Finally, our special thanks go to Mrs Daphne Green for so ably translating rough drafts into an ordered typescript.

How to use this book

This is a practical book, for use in surgery, clinic or ward. It advises when and how to use medication to help people with behavioural and psychological disturbances, whether these are primary mental illnesses or secondary to physical illness. Drug prescriptions are described in the context of the general management of the individual patient. Where possible, treatments are based on securely established fact, otherwise they represent our own experience and what we teach as good practice. The management suggested is not necessarily the only successful way of doing things, but one we can recommend in the present state of knowledge. However, it is based on our belief that careful consideration of the choice, method of introduction and dose schedule of drugs results in better therapeutic results and less toxicity.

In the past, many psychiatrists have been prepared to take great trouble over their psychotherapeutic handling of patients, but used drugs in a fast, indifferent, rule-of-thumb way. They have sometimes been frightened of proper doses or of persisting long enough with medical treatment, and have not learned that understanding chemotherapy can improve the outcomes for their patients. We believe that psychological treatment, informal or formal, must often be combined with drug treatment, in a balanced way, to relieve and to cure.

The book is divided into three parts. The first is the general elementary introduction to the neurobiological background and to psychological and social factors to be borne in mind in good prescribing. It can be read as a whole, or in parts, at any time. The second is a series of short essays on the different psychiatric situations and syndromes usually met, and the third a list of all the drugs currently available in Britain for psychiatric treatment. These two sections work together and have a good deal of cross-referencing. In everyday use one dips into the book by looking up an individual drug through the index of trade and approved names; or uses the symptom index to see what the book says about treatment of a particular symptom or syndrome. Or one can take the patient's diagnosis, read the appropriate management essay and look up the mentioned drugs in the drug list.

While, simply for information, we give the names of all available drugs, we give details about only a few. In each group we discuss one at length that we regard as typical of the group and well established, and in general to be most highly recommended, and follow it with shorter entries on some others of the same group that we regard as useful. But we rarely say anything about the newest drugs, because we think it best to gain experience first with drugs whose advantages, shortcomings and risks have been proved over a long period. When describing side-effects we try to name the commonest and most important first, the lesser ones later; we do not list all the side-effects ever reported because to do so is to raise unnecessary fears and to blur the impact of the important with excessive information about the rare.

This is an elementary book, for beginners in psychiatry, medical students, general practitioners and casualty officers, and perhaps helpful also to nurses, social workers and clinical psychologists. It is not intended as a consultant's guide, or as a review of progress in psychopharmacology. There is deliberately very little about neurotransmitter receptors or the molecular biology of synapses (though there is a little in the first section). While it may be interesting, and a basis for theories and further research, to know that neuroleptics can block dopamine receptors or that tricyclics interfere with re-uptake of transmitter amines released at synapses, this is at present largely irrelevant (at times even misleading) when it comes to treating a human patient. We use the drugs we do on the basis of empirical experience with many patients of different types, and their careful clinical study, and not because of any hypotheses about the nature of mental illnesses.

Our book reports some of this experience. It is in no sense a text of psychopharmacology. That is why, while we describe how to look critically at reports on assessments of new drugs, we do not give details on how to conduct a clinical trial. Everyday practice is our touchstone.

1 Prescribing for psychiatric patients

The use of drugs in psychiatry differs from their use in other branches of medicine in three important ways.

Psychotropic drugs suppress psychological symptoms and morbid behaviour which has no known physical pathology. How drugs do this is unknown. The justification for their use is based entirely on clinical experience. The contrast with the knowledge of disease pathology and drug action which supports drug use in general medicine is striking.

Mental illness interferes with insight, the capacity to view an illness with objectivity and agree the correct treatment. Mental illness may even prevent recognition that an illness exists at all. Impairment of insight, a topic barely relevant to general medical patients, often interferes with understanding the point of medication and adherence to a plan of treatment.

Every individual has a social existence, and disturbances in behaviour and feelings can have enormous repercussions on family, friends and workmates. Therefore, treatment of individuals may harm or help those around them and this must always be borne in mind.

How does this affect the prescribing of psychotropic drugs? Firstly, psychotropic drugs suppress symptoms and are used to tide the patient over until the brain dysfunction, whatever it may be, remits. After some months of use, when a drug such as lithium or chlorpromazine is stopped, the symptoms originally abolished may reappear.

Psychiatric diagnoses depend on groups of symptoms occurring together and have no basis in pathology or aetiology.

So labels such as schizophrenia or neurotic depression cannot imply a single pathological entity or a particular chemotherapy. Although many symptoms of schizophrenia are often suppressed by chlorpromazine, this is not an antischizophrenic drug, and to think so will create prescribing error and poor outcomes for some patients.

Chemotherapy is based on trial and error, on empirical experience, and it is sometimes justifiable to use a psychotropic drug in novel circumstances. This is how effective knowledge has so far been built up, and will be extended. But a consequence is that follow-up of the patient to discover what exactly happened after one week, one month, even one year on the drug is more important in psychiatry than in general medicine. This is how useful personal experience, and general knowledge, grow.

Secondly, patients may find it difficult to believe they are ill, or that a physical agent can help them solve what may appear to them as an emotional problem, or face what seems to them some unpleasant reality. They will need psychological handling to accept a drug. The doctor has to engender confidence and assess how much of the patient's behaviour is personality and how much the disability of illness. For example, was he always a timid, anxious, hypochondriacal person; has illness made him suspicious of everyone, or forgetful? The answers determine what the doctor says and does in explaining the illness and what can be done about it and how a drug or medicine may play a part.

Not only personality, morbid and pre-morbid, but lifestyle must be taken into account. Someone who is worried about chemical pollution of the environment or the risks of drug addiction may need psychotherapeutic persuasion to accept a psychotropic drug, and understanding the individual's particular difficulties is helpful. Drugs with sedative side-effects should not be prescribed to be taken at times which will interfere with driving or work. The regular alcoholic drinkers will not take medicines which they think go poorly with alcohol and, if they cannot be otherwise persuaded to avoid drinking, one should try to arrange a compromise with them rather than abandoning treatment. A man who always takes cheese sandwiches to work will not want a monoamine oxidase inhibitor. Someone on the night shift will not want a drug thrice daily. Very frequently, therefore, psychiatric prescribing is much more than writing the names and doses of drugs on a sheet of paper. It involves a psychotherapy in which the doctor accepts and neutralises the patient's fears, and a choice of drug and a timing of doses to suit the patient's daily routine.

Thirdly, it is always useful to ask oneself, "who has sent this patient to the clinic?", "why is this patient in hospital?", meaning "who has urged or insisted that the patient seek medical help?", because very often relations or workmates, social workers or lawyers or other outside professionals have prompted referral and are expecting some change in the patient. Treatment has therefore to be directed towards them, too. For example, a person who is getting up in the middle of the night and going downstairs to wander about may not complain of insomnia or daytime fatigue, but may be alarming his relatives by his unpredictability, and a hypnotic prescribed to the patient may be primarily to soothe them. Of course, the relatives should be given some explanation of the nature of the illness, and what to expect from it and from the treatment plan, but the drug prescription may take them into account, too.

Psychiatric illness may impair sufferers' self-awareness and knowledge of the impression they make on others, and may also diminish the care they take of themselves and their appreciation of their own interests. Doctors must therefore take on a greater responsibility for their patients, a quasi-parental role, if they are to serve them well, and serve the community in which they live. General practitioners in particular quite commonly leave it to patients to come back to them if they are dissatisfied or not doing well. This will often not do for psychiatric patients; the doctor must give them a definite follow-up appointment (and if it is not kept, check why not, and make another) for a day or two hence, or a week or two, to see whether the prescription has resulted in any changes. It may be important to ask a relative to come to the appointment too (or to phone in some report). The patient may not have taken the medicine, or may say it has done no good, whereas the relative may have noted a striking improvement; or it may have produced new symptoms and the doctor should learn of this.

An important part of the art of practice is knowing when to follow up, how often and for how long, and in what ways. Psychiatric illness in particular is often chronic even though fluctuating in severity or punctuated by long remissions. It is especially important to have some rational plan of when and how to follow it through, and to ask other members of the community, particularly those close to the patient, from time to time to give their impressions of progress.

With psychiatric patients one quite often needs to make a balanced judgement between opposing considerations. Thus psychiatric illness sometimes impairs commonsense and self-care. If left to care for themselves they may fail to do so. How far in respect for the individual and the right to self-determination should one let a patient go, even perhaps to allowing suicide, or should one intervene at some point and complete some kind of treatment? Suppose a young schizophrenic is unable to work or look after himself and is willing to have treatment, but the only drug which helps him back to some semblance of normality carries some risk of causing brain damage: should one prescribe it or not? A woman with a history of several manic–depressive breakdowns is successfully kept free of further breakdowns with lithium carbonate, but wants to be or becomes pregnant. Lithium may cause foetal malformation: should she stop lithium forthwith, and run the risk of further breakdowns (suicidal depression, or reckless excitement, perhaps) or let the foetus carry the risk of cardiac anomaly? We believe each case must be considered individually to balance the various desires and risks against one another, not decided by some rule of thumb 'No' or 'Yes'.

In the next chapters, there are explanations of how drug interactions can occur. In psychiatry some of these interactions are beneficial, some adverse, and they may be overlooked. An example of an apparent beneficial interaction is between chlorpromazine and lithium which together may suppress schizophrenic illness not well controlled by either drug alone. Often two or more drugs have to be prescribed at the same time, and interaction may occur in absorption and metabolism, or at some central intracerebral points. The persistence of metabolites and other effects after a drug has been stopped may influence the actions of the next drug taken.

The art of prescribing includes the following considerations:

(a) the symptoms to be targeted in the short and the long term
(b) age, physical health and circumstances
(c) drugs already taken, including home remedies such as cough cures
(d) the effectiveness, and otherwise, of previous drug treatments
(e) personality and lifestyle
(f) the social setting
(g) the choice of actual drugs, size and schedule of dose
(h) when to review outcome and who should help report it.

Not infrequently the answers to these considerations conflict and do not lead to a logical, ideal drug treatment. For example, an antidepressant may impair driving ability and a commercial driving licence can be suspended, with temporary loss of employment and income. A chronic neurotic may only tolerate conditions at work and earn a salary with the chemical support of an anxiolytic.

Decisions from conflicting evidence are common in medicine. They are best made after discussion with the patient and the patient's relatives or others who have a legitimate interest. Ultimately, however, the doctor, because of his or her technical knowledge and experience, must decide, acting in the best interests of the patient.

In the following chapters "The biological context" deals with relevant pharmaceutical, pharmacological and metabolic aspects of drugs. "Clinical practice" covers some psychological and social points and under the heading "Unexpected results" discusses what to do when treatment unexpectedly fails, or new symptoms appear, and includes idiosyncrasies and the investigation of drug interactions.

2 The biological context

Pharmacology

When a doctor prescribes for a patient who takes the drugs the effects are both pharmacological and psychological. The latter arise because human beings are responsive to their doctors, to their changing social environment, and to their own sensations and expectations, and can be influenced by what the doctor says and does. It is always necessary to try to disentangle the pharmacological from the psychological response in treatment, so as to remain in control of the drugs. Here we are concerned with the physical factors which determine the pharmacological response in the patient. Some affect the difficulty with which the drug in a tablet enters the body and travels in the circulation to enter a well protected brain, others the way it alters the functional balance between different groups of nerve cells. Modern psychotropic drugs have been known for less than 40 years and their discovery has been largely accidental. How to use them safely and effectively has been found by the hard practical experience of treating thousands of patients, made more precise by the pharmaceutical and metabolic considerations described briefly below, and not by any understanding of biochemical mechanisms of drug action. Neurotransmitter studies and theories, though intellectually appealing, have proved so far to have little relevance to clinical practice. Careful detailed observation of what drugs do, singly and in combination, in human beings suffering in differing ways, remains the line of progress in therapeutics.

Language

It will be useful to explain a number of terms used in clinical pharmacology. *Pharmacokinetics* is the study of all the factors which determine the concentration of drug at its site of action, whereas *pharmacodynamics* is the study of mechanisms of action and drug effects. It is the former we are mostly concerned with here. *Bioavailability* is the extent to which less drug reaches the brain in unit time when taken by a patient orally as a pharmaceutical dose than when given in the same quantity of pure drug intravenously.

In trying to understand the relation between size of dose, concentration in the blood and duration of clinical effect, a simple model is often used. The body is assumed to be a single vessel of fluid in which the drug will rapidly disperse, and the *volume of distribution* of a drug is the volume of the imaginary vessel as shown by the diluted plasma level to which the drug falls shortly after its administration and rapid absorption. Elimination of most drugs follows exponential or *first-order kinetics*, that is a constant fraction of the whole in the body is eliminated per unit of time, independent of the actual concentration of the drug. But a few (e.g. phenytoin, alcohol) are eliminated by rather feeble processes, by enzymes present in such small amount that the amount of drug present quickly saturates them. When the enzymes are working thus at maximum pitch, a constant steady quantity of drug is eliminated per unit of time, whatever the body load. This slower process is one of *zero-order kinetics* and its duration depends on the drug concentration. The elimination *half-time*, the time taken to eliminate half the drug administered, is a convenient measure of persistence in the body, which will affect the frequency of dosing. Another measure of this is the *clearance*, the fraction of the total volume of distribution emptied, theoretically, of all drug in unit time.

Measurements of plasma concentrations of a drug at various times after a single intravenous dose can show the elimination kinetics, the volume of distribution and elimination half-time, and thereby indicate what dose, repeated with what frequency, should be used to achieve any chemical concentration in body fluids at any particular time. They are used to establish how to use a drug, especially a new one, but are not needed in everyday practice. *Tolerance* is where a continuing drug effect can only be obtained with increasing doses ('tachyphylaxis' is the very rapid development of tolerance, after only two or three doses). *Dependence* is where there are physical or psychological symptoms on attempted withdrawal. *Drug addiction* is where much time is spent on drug-seeking and drug-taking behaviour, with physical and psychological symptoms on withdrawal.

Bioavailability

Not all tablets or capsules disintegrate easily in the stomach, and not all suspensions have particles of the right size for easy solution or absorption. Different preparations or brands of the same dose of the same drug do not always yield the same amount of drug in the patient. Oral preparations do not keep indefinitely, and many preparations have a limited shelf-life and may deteriorate after their 'use-by' date. Intramuscular injections of the same preparation of the same dose of a drug do not always give the same effect. Choice of muscle, needle position, depth of injection, tissue trauma and blood flow through the muscle influence speed and completeness of absorption. Inactivity and poor circulation, notably in the chronic schizophrenic, the elderly, and the physically ill may slow uptake. A tablet is not all active drug, but contains an excipient which binds together and adds bulk to the tablet and is covered with a coating. An injection has a vehicle; a syrup may have a solvent, a stabiliser and a preservative. Occasionally these supposedly inert substances have unexpected, unwanted effects, producing for example an allergic reaction. (Changing to another brand of the same drug, made up differently, may then avoid these bad effects.) Defects in bioavailability may sometimes explain the failure of a drug to produce the intended response.

Absorption

Some drugs are absorbed from the stomach, others only from a part of the intestine. Delayed gastric emptying may slow the action of intestinally absorbed drugs if taken before a meal, when the pylorus is shut. Some drugs, lithium carbonate for instance, are gastric irritants and best taken with some food. The pH of gastric and intestinal contents, intestinal hurry or delay, the nature of the diet and its digestion, may influence absorption. A partial gastrectomy, malabsorption syndromes, and diarrhoea may alter the speed and completeness with which a drug enters the portal circulation from the gut.

Drugs absorbed from the gastrointestinal tract must pass through the liver and some are at once partly destroyed there ('first-pass metabolism', which may be very large) before distribution to the rest of the body. Others, diazepam for instance, have therapeutically active metabolites produced in the liver. In contrast, drugs given intravenously, intramuscularly, or sublingually are distributed to lung and then to brain and body with a smaller fraction to the liver. By these routes the brain gets a bigger share of the drug than from the same oral dose. Since liquids or syrups are more quickly absorbed than the contents of tablets, they too may give rather more drug to the brain. How a drug is to be taken (by mouth?), in what form (age and brand of tablet?), and how often (once a day?), often need to be considered.

Metabolism

The liver is the chief site of drug metabolism, but lung, gut, kidney and placenta also attack drugs and so do the microflora of the gut (Fig. 1). Liver enzymes that metabolise drugs are reliably increased in quantity, or induced, over a week or more by many substances – tobacco smoke, alcohol, phenytoin, and some psychotropic drugs. Heavy drinkers, and smokers, epileptics and other chronic drug users may therefore need bigger doses of a psychotropic drug than usual if the brain is to get its share. Chlorpromazine and carbamazepine stimulate the liver enzymes that destroy them. Their psychotropic effects sometimes seem to wear off after about two weeks of use because additional enzyme becomes active and the drug is destroyed more quickly. A higher dose is then needed. In contrast, patients with congestive cardiac failure or other cause of limited hepatic blood flow, liver damage, babies with underdeveloped liver function, and the elderly with diminished hepatic performance require smaller doses of psychotropic drugs than the norm for their body weight.

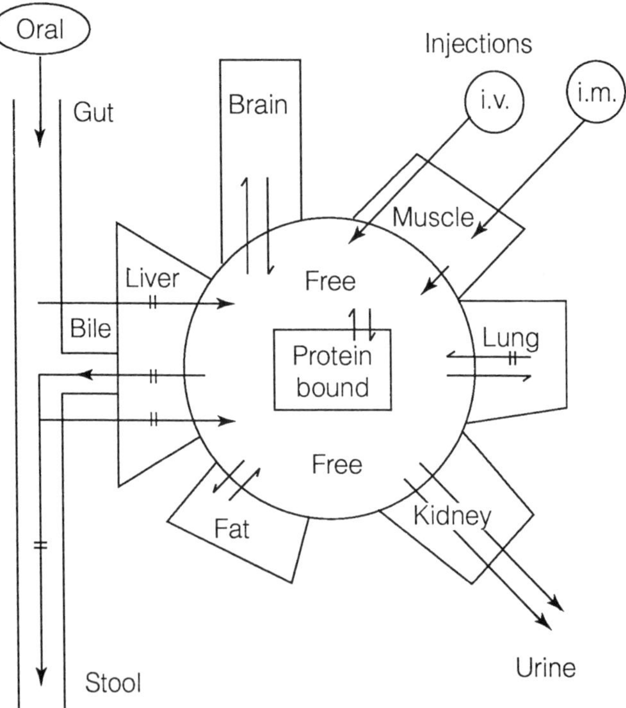

Fig. 1. A diagram of drug metabolism. The circle represents the blood, arrows indicate drug movement, and parallel lines on arrow shaft indicate drug metabolism

Certain steroids, particularly progestogens, which are used in oral contraceptives, inhibit drug metabolism. A female patient taken off 'the pill' may then require more psychotropic drug as metabolism increases. Pregnant women, with their raised progesterone levels, metabolise drugs less effectively during pregnancy. Drugs to be continued through pregnancy may need to be reduced in dose to avoid overdose effects, if they are subject to metabolic destruction, but increased again after labour. Lithium, which is not metabolised, shows an opposite effect: it is excreted more rapidly during pregnancy, and therefore the pregnant woman needs an increased dose, which must be reduced and reset at once in the puerperium. Drug metabolism is sometimes considered in two phases. Phase I involves enzymatic oxidation or reduction, demethylation and hydrolysis: all produce metabolites which are less lipid-soluble, sometimes pharmacologically more active, more often inert. Phase II is conversion of phase I metabolites to glucuronides, sulphates or other conjugates which are very water-soluble and excreted by the kidney. Phase I metabolism becomes impaired in the elderly, but phase II is less affected by ageing.

Entero-hepatic circulation

Drugs of larger molecular size and their metabolites are secreted by the liver into the bile and periodically emptied into the gut, some to be reabsorbed into the blood. This entero-hepatic circulation of drugs results in a reserve of drug and metabolites remaining in bile and gut contents, only some passing out in the faeces. Further, metabolites inactivated by hepatic oxidation may be reactivated by chemical reduction through the activity of intestinal microflora. Reactivated drugs then reappear in the circulation and prolong the pharmacological action. Drugs excreted mainly in the bile and faeces therefore take longer to clear from the body than those excreted in urine. The normality or 'health' of a patient's microflora may influence what happens.

Fat solubility

Many drugs are especially soluble in body fat. Once in the body the drug is shared unequally between the body and brain, the body getting most of it. A fat body gets an even larger share, so the brain gets even less. A child of four has a brain of almost adult size which results in the brain getting a larger share of a dose than an adult brain would. When a drug is first circulating it rapidly enters the brain, but then, if it is lipid-soluble, it is taken up extensively by body fat, and so it is rapidly withdrawn from the brain again. In this case it has a short activity half-life, but a long elimination half-life. Lorazepam is such a drug.

Renal excretion

Some drugs are excreted almost entirely in the urine; lithium is an example. Others are excreted partly in the urine and partly in faeces. Thirty per cent of imipramine and only 10% of thioridazine are lost through the kidneys. Good renal function is essential for clearing many drugs and their metabolites from the body. Poor blood flow through the kidney, as in cardiac failure, or in renal disease as in chronic nephritis, or normally in the infant under one year old, may result in partial or complete failure to clear a drug. Normal doses then have the effect of an overdose. The extreme case is prescribing during renal failure treated by dialysis where the drug is only removed periodically in the dialysate, and has to be prescribed accordingly.

Urinary excretion of drugs that are weak bases or weak acids depends on urine pH, which may vary with diet and exercise. Conditions that favour salt formation also favour drug excretion. Thus a weak base such as amphetamine is rapidly excreted if the urine is strongly acid, since it then forms salts which are not reabsorbed; but if the urine is markedly alkaline, the free un-ionised base diffuses out of the renal tubules back into the blood, and drug action on the brain is much prolonged. The urine can be made acid with doses of ammonium chloride or alkaline with sodium bicarbonate or potassium citrate.

Drugs in the blood

Since samples of circulating blood are easily drawn, measurement of the amount of a drug in the blood is a simple approach to the question of how much drug is reaching the sensitive areas of the brain – provided a sensitive and specific method exists for analysing that drug. It is then possible to correlate the therapeutic and side-effects of the drug with its plasma concentration, provided: (a) the clinical effect follows soon after the drug reaches the brain, (b) it is due directly to the drug and not to some metabolite, and (c) the drug–brain receptor interaction is reversible (for most monoamine oxidase inhibitors it is not).

Thus for phenytoin and for lithium it is possible to find plasma concentrations associated with beneficial effects, and higher concentrations associated with adverse or toxic effects. These concentrations are similar but not identical in different individuals, which gives rise to the idea of a therapeutic range of values for a given population of patients. Low lithium concentrations have had little effect in suppressing the excitement of cohorts of American and British manic patients. (This might not apply to other ethnic groups.) As the lithium concentrations are raised above 0.7 mmol/l different patients respond as higher concentrations are achieved, but raising the level above 1.4 mmol/l has not produced any further benefit, and over 2.0 mmol/l toxic signs appear. Under these circumstances the therapeutic range of lithium for treatment of mania is said to be 0.7–1.4 mmol/l, which means that the vast majority, of Anglo-Americans at least, will be expected to do well on doses producing a plasma level in this range. But one particular individual may only do well at the top of the range (e.g. 1.2 mmol/l), while a second recovers on 0.8 mmol/l, and a third may require 1.0 mmol/l.

Similarly, nortriptyline levels below 50 ng/ml (or 50 μg/l) will effect nothing, and values above 150 ng/ml will do nothing either, except cause side-effects or perhaps even inhibit recovery. This therapeutic range 50–150 ng/ml is sometimes called a therapeutic window.

Anticonvulsants, tricyclics and butyrophenones have been measured in this way. For the first it is a useful guide to successful treatment, for the second the value is controversial, the third a tool of research. One difficulty is that the clinical response (e.g. relief of depression) follows 10 days or more after the establishment of the drug level. What is happening in this time, and how is it related to the quantities of drug arriving over 10 days?

Individual patients differ very considerably in how they absorb and metabolise the same dose of the same drug. In a group all given 100 mg amitriptyline daily on the same schedule there is at least a tenfold difference between the lowest and the highest individual plasma levels obtained. It was, therefore, hoped that blood measurements would guide in deciding clinical dosage for the individual, but this has not on the whole proved possible. Plasma measurements, of course, reveal whether the patient has taken the prescribed drug (though not necessarily in the doses proposed), but they are rather an expensive way of testing compliance. They have been useful in studying drug toxicity (when linked to abnormally high plasma concentrations of drug), and they are valuable in the discovery of drug interactions. For example, when chlorpromazine is added to a steady treatment with imipramine, the plasma concentrations of imipramine and desipramine rise almost at once to much higher levels. This is due to the competitive inhibition in the liver of imipramine metabolism by chlorpromazine, an interaction first discovered from plasma measurements. Many examples are now known where one drug inhibits the metabolism of another, or alternatively speeds up its destruction, and blood measurement has been important in the discovery. This is important, therefore, in the analysis of unusual or unexpected drug responses.

There are two very important points to remember when interpreting measurements of plasma concentration of drugs.

The first is that a blood sample is taken at a moment in time, and the measurement, therefore, applies only to that moment, like a snapshot. Other times of day might yield other values. Therefore, when taking a blood sample always mark the exact time it was drawn, and when comparing samples on different days try always to take them at the same time of day, and always avoid times soon after the actual taking of drug doses. With lithium this is particularly important because lithium is rapidly absorbed, and the plasma level rises rapidly in the next four hours and then falls away exponentially: blood for clinically useful lithium measurement should never normally be drawn within eight hours of a dose, preferably longer.

The second point is that with most drugs (but not lithium) the plasma proteins modify the values the laboratory returns. Most drugs circulate partly dissolved freely in the plasma water, and pharmacologically active, but largely (80–90%) bound reversibly to plasma albumin and pharmacologically inactive when bound. The laboratory reports the total drug in the plasma, free plus protein-bound, and unfortunately the latter is subject to hidden changes. If the plasma albumin is low, as in liver disease, the protein-bound drug will be low and the total concentration will be low, but the pharmacological action just the same because the free drug concentration is the same. Or the albumin may be normal but its binding capacity for the drug being measured may be low, either because of competitive interference from another drug (very important when using two or more anticonvulsants in epileptic treatment) or because of metabolic interference – the binding is altered in uraemia, diabetes, ketosis, and starvation. Or the binding protein itself can be increased in some chronic inflammatory conditions (Crohn's disease) or after trauma or surgery, and then bound drug will be high, total drug level high, yet free drug perhaps only just adequate. So plasma drug concentrations offer many pitfalls, and are not quite the excellent guide to drug therapy that was first hoped.

Babies and drugs

Many drugs cross the placenta. The baby of a mother taking lithium may be born with hypothyroidism caused by the lithium; a morphine-dependent woman may produce a drug-dependent infant. With some drugs the chief risk may be to cause an anomaly of development, which is then chiefly in the first three months of foetal life, when anatomy is decided, and not thereafter. In deciding whether or not to give such drugs during pregnancy the time in the pregnancy is clearly important, but also it is necessary to weigh the pros and cons of treatment for both mother and for foetus and not just for the one of them.

Drugs also appear in breast milk, in proportion to their free concentration (not bound to protein, or total) in the maternal circulating plasma. Therefore, drugs like phenothiazines and tricyclics which are mostly protein-bound are of little import, but lithium, which is free, can matter. These considerations may contraindicate breast-feeding, unless the maternal drug can reasonably be stopped. Infants in the first year of life have poor renal and hepatic function so that clearance of drug is slow at this time.

If a woman has to take drugs during pregnancy remember that renal blood flow (and hence urinary excretion) increases at this time, but that the increased progesterone secretion suppresses hepatic metabolism of drugs. Drug dosage may need to be adjusted in the light of those facts, and readjusted in the puerperium.

Drug interactions

The simultaneous prescription of more than one drug is often necessary. However, drugs may interfere with each other's absorption from the gut, binding in the plasma, excretion in the urine, metabolism in the liver and effects in the brain. Some examples illustrate the point. Carbamazepine, like barbiturates, stimulates liver enzymes that destroy imipramine, phenytoin and other drugs, and may reduce the clinical effects of these drugs. Monoamine oxidase inhibitors block phenytoin metabolism and may cause phenytoin toxicity. Orphenadrine stimulates the liver enzymes that destroy chlorpromazine, diminishing the levels of chlorpromazine, as well as interacting in the brain to diminish its effects on the extrapyramidal system. In contrast chlorpromazine prevents the liver metabolism of imipramine. Some drug interactions are clinically useful. Lithium and thioridazine, for instance, may be more effective in schizophrenia when given together than either alone. Lithium and imipramine together may suppress depressive illness, when neither alone will do so. More such interactions remain to be recognised.

Drugs in the brain

Psychotropic drugs act at a molecular or subcellular level. They combine with receptors, which may be molecules of an enzyme or part of a membrane, altering porosity, configuration, ability to combine with a natural neurotransmitter, and in other ways. A drug may have a number of such actions but one may be clinically more important than the others. The clinical effects of a drug can only be rarely related to its molecular actions (e.g. drugs combining with dopamine receptors cool mania). What happens in a brain slice or an acute animal preparation is less complex than what may happen over a period in the whole brain of man. A brief account of brain structure will clarify this.

The brain is a vast assembly of neurones of different sizes and designs which communicate with each other by releasing small amounts of neurotransmitters when excited. Each neurone has branching threads or dendrites extending from its cell body, and a thicker longer axon which also may divide into several filaments. Each axon ends in 500 or more terminal buttons which make contact with specialised surfaces on other neurones. Each button and its contact point form a synapse. One neurone may have hundreds of synapses. When an electrical impulse arrives at a button, neurotransmitter is released and passes across the synaptic cleft to combine with receptor molecules on the next neurone. If enough buttons release appropriate transmitter to activate enough receptor areas, the post-synaptic neurone becomes excited and passes a new impulse along its axon. Each synapse releases one type of neurotransmitter, but all the buttons from one neurone do not necessarily release the same substance. A single neurone can be stimulated or inhibited by more than one kind of neurotransmitter.

Receptors

The receptor areas (e.g. of membranes) are important as the origin of some of the adaptability of the central nervous system. The large receptor molecules are being continually synthesised and then broken down again, so their number at synapses is not necessarily constant. The cell makes them in relation to the neurotransmitter stimulation it receives. When there is little transmitter making contact, the number of receptors is increased so that the neurone responds to low transmitter as powerfully as it would have done to an ordinary transmitter level. When transmitter release is high, the receptors diminish so that the response in time comes down to an ordinary level again in spite of the excess transmitter.

Thus, when haloperidol blocks the access of dopamine to its receptor the number of receptors goes up, as shown by the development of supersensitivity to the action of a dopamine agonist. When a tricyclic antidepressant prevents noradrenaline reuptake and floods a synapse with the amine, the neurone responds with a decrease (down-regulation) in the number of β-adrenoceptors. These changes take several weeks for completion, and, interestingly, lithium has been shown to prevent dopamine supersensitivity arising, and also the increase of β-receptors when noradrenaline is depleted in response to reserpine. But it is not yet clear how this can produce therapeutic benefit, or permanent change in the nervous system; nor is its significance for the pathology of a psychosis clear.

Many substances act as neurotransmitters. Some are amines such as acetylcholine, serotonin, noradrenaline or dopamine; others are amino acids such as gamma amino-butyric acid (GABA) and glycine; and others still are peptides, substance P and endorphins for instance. More await discovery.

To the unaided eye, and even more so under the microscope, the brain has a complex anatomical structure. Neurones are arranged in small or large groups, possibly delimited by groups of glial cells which may create semi-permeable boundaries around them or special local chemical environments. Axons may run for long distances connecting one part of the brain with another, and the kinds of neurotransmitters released vary from region to region. The brain shows a complex chemical patterning as the counterpart of the anatomical pattern, although distinct from it. Functionally the structure can be considered at the levels of the individual neurone and the neuronal group. In the single cell neurotransmitter is synthesised and stored. When a nerve impulse reaches a terminal button, transmitter is released from storage granules into the synaptic cleft. There, some combines reversibly with receptors, some is destroyed by enzymes and quite a large part is reabsorbed into the button by a metabolically driven transport process.

Psychotropic drugs may work by interfering with these processes. Imipramine inhibits the button's reuptake process for noradrenaline, and to a lesser extent for serotonin. Imipramine also blocks acetylcholine receptors. Haloperidol blocks dopamine receptors. Physostigmine inhibits choline-esterase which destroys acetylcholine. Phenelzine inhibits the monoamine oxidase that destroys released serotonin.

Drug concentrations at different brain sites are not necessarily the same, nor are all receptors for one transmitter identical, so a drug may not have an equal effect at all its action sites. For example, dopamine synapses are not all equally blocked by haloperidol. Different receptors for the same neurotransmitter are numbered -1,-2, alpha or beta, etc. They are distinguished by differences in their responses to a range of similar drugs.

Drugs act on other parts of the neurone besides the neurotransmitter mechanisms. Barbiturates inhibit elements of the energy-producing machinery of the cell, and phenytoin modifies intracellular control of electrolyte transport. Much less is known about drug effects on neuronal groups. Neurones appear to be organised into functional networks which control, for example, the release of pituitary hormones, the setting of body temperature, sleep, arousal, the regulation of body weight and fluid content. Neurological disease may reveal some of this organisation by disturbing it. Parkinsonism appears to be due to a deficiency of the neurotransmitter dopamine. Stimulating the production of dopamine or the release of more dopamine with L-dopa improves the symptoms and signs. But improvement can be produced by benzhexol, which blocks acetylcholine receptors. So the disorder is due not only to lack of dopamine but an imbalance between dopamine and acetylcholine activities, at the least. Huntington's disease appears to result from GABA deficiency. However, phenothiazines which block dopamine receptors may reduce the abnormal movements, which suggests the condition must in part be caused by a GABA–dopamine imbalance.

The reticular activating system in the centre of the brain receives a sensory input which excites it: the consequent increased arousal may first lead to alertness, then to pathological excitement. One action of phenothiazines appears to be a preferential blockade of some of this sensory input. It has been proposed that patients with schizophrenia have an abnormally increased sensitivity to this sensory input. By blocking the input chlorpromazine reduces arousal and makes for more healthy behaviour. This hypothesis is of a higher order of organisation, involving a functional anatomical unit, than the dopamine hypothesis of the cause of schizophrenia which suggests that schizophrenia results from an abnormality of dopamine receptors, a molecular-level concept. Theories about how drugs work have concentrated on their immediate effects. But it is now realised that the brain has powers of adjusting to the chemical stimulation of drugs over a period of weeks or months. Improved understanding of this phenomenon may help advance knowledge about the treatment and the pathology of disease.

Side-effects are equally part of a drug's action, simply unwanted consequences, just as weeds may equally be flowering plants, but unwanted in a garden. Side-effects result from the drug's action both in the central nervous system and elsewhere. Imipramine, for example, causes a dry mouth. The dryness is due partly to cholinergic blockade in the salivary glands preventing secretion of saliva, and partly to a central inhibitory action on the nuclei of the medulla controlling salivation. The action of imipramine in preventing nocturnal bed-wetting in children may result from one or all of the following effects: direct anaesthetic action on the bladder lessening bladder irritability; a metabolic antidiuretic action reducing urine volume; changes in synaptic transmission in the spinal cord altering bladder reflexes; a central action changing sleep pattern. The complexity of a drug's activity illustrates the need to remember that the central nervous system is more than the cerebral cortex and immediate subcortical structures of primary interest to the psychiatrist. The mid-brain, hind-brain and spinal cord contain the same synaptic machinery as the cerebral cortex. Psychotropic drugs can act at all levels of the central nervous system.

Neurones are like the letters of the alphabet. It is their arrangement in functional sequences and groups which gives them meaning. Breaking the code is going to depend on a combined behavioural and neurological analysis of drug actions in health and disease at many levels of central nervous organisation. Mania can be controlled with haloperidol, blocking dopamine transmission, or with physostigmine, improving acetylcholine transmission by inhibiting the esterase that destroys it, or with lithium which does neither of these. What neuronal network does this imply? It is because we are so ignorant of the neurological bases of psychotic symptoms that the molecular actions of drugs tell us very little about their clinical effects. Neurotransmitter theory is so far of little clinical relevance: antidepressant drugs with chiefly noradrenergic action seem just as effective as antidepressant drugs that are serotonergic. Another consequence of this ignorance is that diagnoses, in terms of drug therapeutic response, are dubious. A third is that, with so little yet known, a certain amount of experimenting with unlikely treatments is justified when the conventional ones have failed. But it ought to be done systematically and recorded. Even if no new drugs are discovered in the next ten years, new uses will be found for the existing ones and the precision in their use greatly improved.

Finding new drugs

Psychotropic drugs have been discovered mostly by accident and clinical observation rather than planned development. Chlorpromazine, first introduced as an antihistamine, was used as part of an anaesthetic cocktail before successful trial as a sedative in mania in 1954. Then it was tried in other mental disorders and found to be useful in schizophrenia as well. This discovery stimulated the synthesis of many other phenothiazines. One hundred and thirty-eight are listed in Usdin & Efron's *Psychotropic Drugs and Related Compounds* (1972), although only 60 or so have been prescribed. If there seem to be even more it is because of the many trade names for the same drug around the world. Chlorpromazine has had over 70. Except in potency, duration of action and side-effects the newer phenothiazines show no substantial advance on chlorpromazine.

Kuhn in *Discoveries in Biological Psychiatry* (Ayd & Blackwell, 1970, pp. 205–207) describes how he discovered the antidepressant action of imipramine. Imipramine was sent to him as a substitute for chlorpromazine. He decided to try it on other disorders than schizophrenia and found its effectiveness in endogenous depression. The discovery of the sedative action of benzodiazepines was more accidental (Ayd & Blackwell,

1970). A research chemist in a drug company tested substances, which he had made for his PhD in organic chemistry 20 years previously, for pharmacological activity. They had none. He made some more of the same series and one turned out to be hypnotic and sedative. It also turned out to be a different substance from that planned because the chemical reactions of synthesis had introduced an unexpected molecular rearrangement. The substance had its first clinical trial on geriatric patients. They became ataxic on the larger doses prescribed and interest evaporated. A second trial, using smaller doses on neurotic out-patients, proved encouraging and chlordiazepoxide, ancestor of the benzodiazepines, started on the road to acceptance.

A chemist synthesises a new substance. Pharmacologists show it has biological activity in tests on blood pressure, temperature control, movement, problem-solving, aggressiveness, sleeping time, and so on, of mice, rats, guinea pigs, monkeys. Toxicologists define the safe limits for ingestion, measure metabolism and speed of excretion. The drug is tested on a few healthy volunteers, then on a few patients with the symptoms someone supposes it might suppress. If after this the drug still seems promising, clinicians test it further on other disorders and at varying dosages. Because of species differences and the effects of illness there is no substitute for the study of the drug in the sick human.

At this stage reports of successful use may appear in the medical press. A pharmaceutical company may decide to launch the drug with an advertising campaign, but before this the drug must be licensed by the government for prescribing. How will you decide whether to try the new drug? The drug company will claim it is more potent, faster, with fewer side-effects and less toxicity than the comparable drugs you already use. The claims will be backed by facts such as animal pharmacology and enzyme chemistry, which really do not matter to the doctor, and clinical reports which do. The clinician can assess the value of this clinical information under the following headings.

By their authority

A report from a scientist of standing, working in a hospital of repute, published in a peer-review journal, is more credible than one from A. Noodle of St Blanket's writing in the Proceedings of the North Cowville Medical Society. Noodle may have the truth, but one wonders whether he had time and facilities to do the work properly and why he hasn't published in a better journal.

By the quality of study

Assess the facts reported in the paper. Are the patients who received the drug clinically recognisable by description, or simply tucked inside some diagnostic parcel? Have the authors seen the patients themselves, or left their assessment to nurses, or to a computer? Are the dose levels of the drug correct? What is the evidence for compliance? Did the treatment go on long enough? What about side-effects? What of the patients who dropped out of treatment? What environmental factors might have played a part in producing good results?

A claim for the effectiveness of a drug is more credible for a well defined syndrome of hitherto poor prognosis. When chlorpromazine was first given to psychotic patients, living in hospital for years and incapable of conversation or organised activity, the results were impressive. Most observers were convinced of the great discovery. With imipramine the situation was different. Depression, a wider diagnostic term than schizophrenia, tends to remit spontaneously or improve with non-specific care and placebo. It was correspondingly more difficult to assess the value of imipramine.

By clinical trial

Credibility increases as favourable reports appear from many sources over a lengthy period. This is the drug's probationary phase. Clinicians are finding out how to use it, looking for drawbacks and virtues. The drug may have a different use from that predicted. Toxicity may appear on long-term use. Advantages over existing drugs may be slight. Effectiveness may appear only when the drug is combined with another. But if, after uncontrolled trials, the drug seems to offer something, though how much is uncertain, the phase of the controlled trial is entered.

A controlled trial is an experiment to see if a treatment influences the course of a disease beneficially. Most commonly a series of patients having the same disease, or fitting the same diagnostic criteria in their symptoms and history, are secretly split into two groups. This can be done at the start, if enough cases are available, or sequentially by allotting new cases to one or the other group randomly (and secretly). Both groups are treated alike except in one respect: only one receives the drug under trial, and the other gets an identical-seeming dummy capsule or tablet. Then the outcome for each patient is assessed at one, two, four weeks, etc., and the two groups compared: is there a difference between them? Less satisfactorily, the second or placebo group, which ordinarily gets the dummy tablet, is sometimes given instead some standard drug, for comparison of outcome with the new one under trial. A true placebo group is important to show the measure of spontaneous improvement, likely in some of any group of patients. Without it spontaneous change is ignored, and the differences between recovery in the two groups made smaller and more difficult to measure.

Sometimes the trial has a cross-over design. Groups A and B receive their separate treatments for, say, four or eight weeks, and then the prescriptions are exchanged. A takes B's drug, and B A's for a further four or eight weeks, change of symptoms being monitored regularly from time to time. The trouble with this is that many drugs continue to produce effects long after they have been stopped, and it is not practicable to allow group A much of a 'washout' period before starting on B's treatment, or vice versa. The second half of the drug trial is therefore studying patients already differently altered (even if invisibly so) from their state in the first half.

A controlled trial considers the following points.

(a) What is the disease being treated? In psychiatry it is usually difficult to be sure that a group of patients with similar symptoms have the same underlying condition. There is no Wassermann reaction, or electrocardiogram or blood glucose determination to serve as a test. Patients referred to a psychiatric ward may differ from area to area, so that the population from which the controlled trial draws cases is not always typical in severity or duration of symptoms, or in tendency to remit. However, Research Diagnostic Criteria (Spitzer *et al*, 1978) have been established and accepted internationally, grouping patients together in terms of a cluster of symptoms. Unfortunately, this does not mean that these groups have a single pathology; but it is helpful in detecting improvement in symptoms.

(b) What is the treatment? What dose is used, how often, for how long? How are different individuals given different doses, which they will need because of individual differences in metabolism, without spoiling the blindness? What about the non-drug part of the treatment?

(c) What is an effect? How is this measured? How many different effects are possible? Is it global recovery that is being examined, or change of symptoms? Who did the measuring, and what was their motivation? Could they have been indifferent or careless in their observations? Rating scales – a list of questions asking about the presence and rough severity of symptoms – have been developed and validated for assessing the severity of a depressive illness or manic attack or the impairment of social adjustment, and so on, and can be used to compare the improvement of patients (particularly groups of patients) subjected to different drug regimes. They can answer questions about the speed and completeness of cure or symptom suppression with drug A or B as compared with placebo improvement, but they are usually not sensitive to the full range of the individual's symptoms and behaviour (nor originally intended to be) and therefore are unsuitable for detecting short-term detailed changes in aspects of the individual's state.

(d) What is the sample size? How many patients were in

the trial, and for how long, and what happened to those who dropped out? How were the dropouts dealt with statistically?

(e) Even statistically significant differences between treated and untreated groups can arise by chance, although this may be unlikely. Nowadays it is very difficult to find patients for controlled trials who have not already had some treatment in the preceding four or eight weeks: this recent treatment may leave effects which interact in an unsuspected way with the trial treatment. Double-blind trials, therefore, need careful critical scrutiny. It should be clear what question they have been designed to answer and evident that it is reliably conducted to answer this question. Trials which try to answer a number of questions at once are usually faulty.

(f) A one-person drug trial is sometimes useful, and avoids some of the pitfalls of the usual group trial (but answers a different question). A single patient is treated first with drug A for a period then with drug B, or placebo, for another period and then back and forth again, the change-over times being blind to patient and staff (both drugs being in identical capsules for the trial) and the patient's symptoms regularly assessed. Drug interactions can be a difficulty here.

Be careful of accepting too readily the conclusions of double-blind trials. A careful trial with conclusions precisely drawn is an inestimable guide to the use of a drug, for the syndrome considered in the trial, for the doses of drug used in the trial, and for the time the drug was used in the trial. In the long run, however, clinical experience, the systematic observation of the results of drug treatment on thousands of patients, decides the fate of a drug.

References

AYD, F. L. & BLACKWELL, B. (eds) (1970) *Discoveries in Biological Psychiatry*. Philadelphia: Lippincott.

SPITZER, R. L., ENDICOTT, J. & ROBINS, E. (1978) Research diagnostic criteria. Rationale and reliability. *Archives of General Psychiatry*, **35**, 773–782.

USDIN, E. & EFRON, D. H. (1972) *Psychotropic Drugs and Related Compounds* (2nd edn). Oxford: Pergamon.

3 Clinical practice

The fact that a drug has been prescribed is no guarantee that the patient has actually fetched the tablets from a pharmacy, or taken them, or taken them in the number and the frequency instructed. In hospital, nurses sometimes withhold doses. Mistakes in administration of drugs occur, patients getting too much, too little or someone else's prescription. Furthermore, some patients who seem to accept the prescribed treatment may secretly palm and throw away their tablets, or hide them in their mouths and secretly spit them out. This is why liquid preparations may be more effective than tablets, and injections surer still.

Whenever a drug seems to fail or to produce unusual results, it is wise to check that it has in fact been taken as instructed. Look at the tablet bottle, ask the patient and the nurse directly, remember that urine tests or blood level measurements exist for some drugs.

Complaints of side-effects result at least as often for psychological as they do for pharmacological reasons. That is often the reason when the patient is upset after only one or two doses, and especially when the dose is small.

True physical sensitivities are rare, psychological sensitivities common. Psychological sensitivities may take the form of anxiety, preoccupation with bodily perceptions, mistrust of doctor or nurse, exaggerated ideas about 'drugs' and their risks, for instance poisoning, addiction, loss of self-control. The doctor must be alive to the patient's attitude to his own body, to his mistrust, to his view of tablets and medicines, if necessary bringing his feelings into open discussion, and possibly modifying the treatment plan if feelings are strong. Confidence is created by giving patients time, showing concern for them and asking about their family and work situation in relation to their illness. It means being unhurried, calm, sincere and confident. The patient who has confidence in the doctor will tolerate the experience of many side-effects without complaint and they may be discovered only on direct inquiry.

It is usually helpful to explain to patients in simple language what each drug is supposed to do for them and the logic of its use, and to add something about the commoner side-effects and what they mean. How this is done must be suited to the intelligence and previous knowledge of the individual patient, and take into account obsessional or hypochondriacal tendencies.

On the positive side, the patient's confidence, suggestibility, belief in the potency of a remedy, which may depend in part on its striking colour or bitter taste, acceptance of the doctor's 'gift' of tablets as symbolic or magical, involving concern or love, the prestige of medical knowledge, and so on, just as much as pharmacology, are factors in the good effect of treatment. Patients will complain of side-effects, or indeed get better, when treated with tablets without any active drug within them. This placebo effect may add to the pharmacological effect where an active drug is also used. The overall effectiveness of treatment, therefore, depends very much on creating the right psychological conditions as well as prescribing the right drug in the right dose.

Two of the commonest reasons for poor results in drug treatment are inadequate dosage, and failure to go on long enough. Frequent newspaper criticism of overprescribing, or of turning people into zombies, persuades doctors to prescribe too little. Some patients try to control their own treatment and demand changes of dose or drug. The doctor should be the technical expert here, with enough clinical knowledge not to be diverted from assessment of the seriousness of the illness, and the pharmacological measures it requires.

Points to remember

Work with a few established drugs and know them well

Know the use of a few drugs thoroughly rather than a large list superficially. Drugs with dose range, side-effects, contraindications and interactions known from extensive use in clinical practice are likely to be better suited for the patient than newly launched drugs with limited experience.

Avoid prescribing more than one drug of the same chemical class at the same time

There is usually no clinical advantage giving, say, amitriptyline with imipramine, or chlorpromazine with trifluoperazine. Treatment is complicated needlessly, patient and nurse burdened with extra tablets. Increase a dose, rather than add a second drug for fear of exceeding some recommended maximum of the first.

If a drug fails, change to one of a different chemical group

When a drug fails, change to a drug from a different group. If amitriptyline does not relieve depression, try a monoamine oxidase inhibitor rather than another tricyclic.

Prescribing 'as required' (p.r.n.) can be risky

Prescribing 'as required' is potentially dangerous because staff who may not have the appropriate clinical or pharmacological knowledge are authorised to give unlimited extra doses of potentially toxic and interacting drugs. The best practice for discretionary medication is written instructions limiting the number of repetitions and their duration, for example, "Repeat dose once, if needed, any night in next five".

Do not prescribe more than three psychotropic drugs at once

Every symptom does not have to be treated, and attempting to do so can result in excessive prescribing. A large number of medicines is a burden to patient, relative and nurse. Errors of dose and timing are more likely to occur and error disrupts the regular timetable of medication. More drugs increase the chance of drug interactions.

Hypnotics may not be necessary to control insomnia

The extra prescription of a hypnotic to control sleeplessness is usually avoidable by giving sedative tricyclics and phenothiazines.

Time tablet-taking to suit the patient's lifestyle

Prescribing a drug to be taken three times a day can become an unthinking habit. Perhaps the drug can be given once a day at a convenient and easily remembered time such as going to bed, for example with tricyclic antidepressants. Dose-related side-effects are more likely with the midday dose because it is so close to the early morning dose. Lunch-time medication tends to be omitted by people at work who forget in the press of the day's events or are embarrassed taking tablets in public. People who work unusual hours (transport drivers, market porters, post-office staff, shift workers) may need advice about timing. People who like cheese sandwiches for lunch will resent monoamine oxidase inhibitors (see p. 155). Those who insist on drinking alcohol will need counsel on when to take their drugs.

Do not reject drugs too soon as ineffective

Prescribe a big enough dose for long enough to be sure a drug has failed before stopping. Phenelzine, for instance, should be tried for four weeks up to 90 mg daily before rejection. Dose response cannot be predicted accurately but it can be found from trial and observation. The discovery of an effective drug and its optimal dose is of such tremendous importance to a patient with a lifetime of chronic or recurring illness that months of careful trial of drugs is justified.

Women may become pregnant

Psychotropic drugs may harm the developing foetus. Before prescribing inquire about the last menstrual period and the patient's intentions about getting pregnant.

The pregnant

A depressive illness or an attack of mania or schizophrenia during pregnancy can be devastating for the mother and potentially a serious threat to the well-being and sometimes life of the unborn child. Where there is a serious risk of a mental breakdown, the prophylactic use of a tricyclic antidepressant, of lithium, or of a phenothiazine may become necessary. Psychotropic drugs may increase the risk of congenital deformities in the baby. Such abnormalities occur in at least 1–2% of pregnancies anyway, with no known cause. Animal experiments with drugs sometimes suggest teratogenicity, but because the experiments are not on humans, and usually with high doses of drugs, such suggestions have to be regarded with reserve. Only human experience of the drug, with careful collection of statistics over a long period, can be the true guide. However, it is fair to say that if the commonly used psychotropic drugs increase the risk of damage to the foetus they do not do so to a great extent, on present knowledge. This small risk must be balanced against the consequences of serious mental illness to the mother and her family. Remember that a drug is likely to be more of a risk for the foetus in higher dosage, and during the first three months of foetal life.

As drug metabolism may be altered during pregnancy, adjust dosage in the pregnant, and readjust in the puerperium.

Infants

Most drugs cross the placental barrier, and also appear in breast milk. The neonate may show withdrawal symptoms if its mother is dependent on opiates or alcohol. The infant may be limp or even goitrous if she takes lithium, but these effects are temporary and cause no lasting harm. Even though the amounts of drug in milk may not be great, the neonate up to about one year old has less than a child or adult in the way of liver hydroxylating enzymes to destroy active drugs, and poor renal function as well. Drugs tend to persist in its body. On present knowledge the doses of phenothiazines, tricyclic antidepressants, anticonvulsants and hypnotics administered to babies in the breast milk of mothers on these drugs are unimportant. Where the mother is taking doses of lithium or diazepam, however, the baby may be affected, and therefore breast feeding is better avoided.

The elderly

As people age they enter a new phase of medical management. Growing old means metabolic impairment often aggravated by chronic disease. Kidneys no longer excrete so well, livers no longer metabolise so fast. Small doses of drugs consequently last longer and exert larger effects. The ageing brain becomes more sensitive to some drugs, benzodiazepines and anti-Parkinsonian drugs especially. These changes occur at different ages for different people and at different rates for different drugs, but are particularly marked in the very old. Older people may have multiple diseases and multiple prescribing, often from two or more sources. They have therefore a much greater tendency than the young to toxic reactions, accidental overdosing, and drug interactions.

Dietary indiscretions, constipation, and inactivity may also have excessive effects on well-being.

Ageing also means psychological impairment. Impaired memory and concentration cause instructions about drugs to be forgotten or muddled. If in charge of their own medication the treatment plan must be simple: few drugs, preferably no more than three, taken on a regular, easily remembered schedule, linked to the fixed points of the day – at meals or when going to bed for instance. Out-patients need written instructions of which medicines to take and when to take them. As a check, have them bring back unused medication from previous prescriptions. A relative, friend, community nurse or warden may be able to take some responsibility for giving the drugs when there is doubt about competence. Complications may arise from self-medication with analgesics, aperients, drugs from the last illness or even from someone else. Psychiatric disorder in the elderly person, especially acute brain syndrome, often results from taking too much prescribed and non-prescribed drugs.

Insomnia with a request for hypnotics is such a common problem in the care of the elderly that a special comment is required. First, find out if the complaint can be treated by simple measures before prescribing a hypnotic. Some lonely old people go to bed in the early evening and get five or six hours' sleep before their 'insomnia' begins, or an after-lunch nap is prolonged, so find out the hours they spend in bed asleep, or trying to sleep, and get independent confirmation. Less time in bed, doing interesting things which require some activity, may give better sleep. Improved bedroom comfort such as correct temperature, quiet, and pillows at the right height, help to promote sleep. Sometimes diet is the culprit. Too much coffee causes excessive arousal by bed-time. Too much fluid during the day can result in repeated waking with a full bladder. Too much food of the wrong kind causes indigestion. Constipation can lead to restlessness.

Medical problems also interfere with sleep. Proper attention to pain, breathlessness, coughing, frequency and the correct timing of diuretic tablets may result in improved sleep.

If a hypnotic has to be used, give small doses and look out for unwanted effects. Be prepared to try several different preparations and aim for an early trial without hypnotics again, because the need for them may vary over time and with changing circumstances. Chloral hydrate preparations, nitrazepam and promazine are all useful in doses about half the size for a younger adult. Short-acting benzodiazepines such as triazolam or temazepam can also be effective while minimising hangover. Avoid barbiturates and long periods on benzodiazepines. However, for patients who have already taken barbiturates or benzodiazepines for a very long time without increasing doses the sensible and humane course may be to continue the prescription. The alternative will be an unhappy patient and possibly withdrawal fits or a psychosis.

Excessive night sedation is dangerous. It causes mental dulling, mental confusion, incontinence, restlessness, wandering, especially at night but sometimes by day, and impairment of balance with a risk of falling. Chest infections are more likely in the heavily sedated.

Unexpected results

No effect

Failure to show any response may be due to 'non-adherence' or 'non-compliance'. The patient has simply not taken the tablets, or taken them irregularly or in less than the prescribed dose. Many patients will admit this on direct kindly questioning, or their relatives will. Otherwise a short period of in-patient nursing observation may be needed to be sure. Measurements of drug plasma levels, if available, may help. Of course, the prescribed dose may have been too little, or even too much, or the illness is truly not susceptible to the drug. But there must be sound evidence that the patient has taken the drug before such an important conclusion is reached.

New symptoms

New mental or physical symptoms other than usual side-effects may appear, particularly after 48 hours, or at around 10 days, or late in the course of chronic treatment. The important question is to decide if the symptoms result from idiosyncrasy, that is, some individual variation of metabolism or unusual immunological response (allergy). If it is, continuing the drug may be dangerous, and it may be impossible ever to give it again. It can be a serious matter if a patient with recurrent depressions or a schizophrenic illness cannot have the clinical benefits of a tricyclic antidepressant or a phenothiazine because of the risks of idiosyncratic response. Therefore, it is important to collect satisfactory evidence before condemning a drug.

Unexpected results have many possible causes. The symptoms may be those of toxic overdosage, taken by mistake or design, or resulting from a dispensing or nursing error. Alternatively, the patient may be intolerant of a usually safe dose of the drug because of an inability to metabolise it normally. That may happen because of an individual metabolic difference, or because some other drug taken at the same time interferes with normal metabolism. Attention to the dose or to the other drugs may put matters right. There may be a coincident onset of a physical illness, which makes the patient intolerant of his usual dose, or produces symptoms such as vomiting or diarrhoea which are mistaken for a toxic reaction.

The idiosyncrasy may not be due to the drug you have prescribed but to some other drug the patient has taken, or even to food. For example, bronchospasm can result from aspirin sensitivity; urticarial rash and fever can be produced by crabmeat. Remember that an allergic idiosyncrasy is sometimes to the coating of a tablet, or to the excipient or vehicle and not to the active drug itself. The idiosyncrasy may be metabolic, for example agranulocytosis with chlorpromazine, or allergic such as cholestatic jaundice, also with chlorpromazine.

The symptoms of idiosyncrasy may include:

(a) in the skin: purpura, urticaria, maculopapular rash, exfoliative dermatitis (eczema)
(b) in the lung: bronchospasm
(c) in the kidney: albuminuria, haemoglobinuria, signs of oliguria and nephritis
(d) in the liver: jaundice
(e) in the blood: sudden drop in platelets, red cells or white cell count (agranulocytosis)
(f) a sudden rise in temperature, with joint pains, swollen glands, and urticaria, 8–10 days after starting may be due to serum sickness, from excess drug antigen reacting with antibody.

What to do in cases of suspected idiosyncrasy

Stop the suspected drug: stop all drugs if that is feasible. Take 10 ml blood and deep-freeze the serum for possible later immunological study. Take a careful drug and chemical history, not only what a doctor has prescribed but what nurses have given or the patient taken of his own accord, for instance proprietary medicines, and what foods, drinks, or industrial chemicals the patient has encountered.

The advice and help of physician, dermatologist and clinical pathologist should be sought. Treatment with corticosteroids may be needed to help the patient over the damage. Blood and urine tests may be needed. Skin tests (prick and scratch or patch) may be advisable to confirm the existence of hypersensitivity.

There may be a possibility of desensitisation. Idiosyncrasy established to one major tranquilliser, for instance, does not ban all. If the patient's psychiatric state requires drug treatment, start cautiously with another phenothiazine, small doses at first, slowly increasing, with daily monitoring of skin and temperature and twice-weekly blood counts and urine analyses until four weeks have passed.

Do not forget to report this drug reaction to the Committee on Safety of Medicines, Freepost, London SW8 5BR.

Look out for these

Unusual reactions can be idiosyncratic, due to an individual's metabolic abnormality or organic pathology, or an acquired allergy. But many are simply rarely observed side-effects, caused perhaps by an over-rapid rise to high drug dose in treatment, or by an over-rapid drug withdrawal, outpacing the central nervous system's capacity to adapt biochemically. Others are the signs of interaction with another drug in the therapy. But some reports of unusual reactions are frankly mistaken: the reactions are not due to a psychotropic drug at all but to a missed organic illness, or to some other chemical with which the patient is in contact, possibly self-prescribed. This is why unusual reactions should be investigated pathologically, in the fullest possible way (including a post-mortem if the patient has died), instead of jumping to some guessed conclusion. A review (Kellam, 1987) of 67 cases of supposed neuroleptic malignant syndrome in the literature drew attention to data suggesting that coincident physical illness such as pulmonary infection or embolism, or myoglobinuria with renal failure, or some febrile sickness could have accounted for the symptoms in 53 of the patients. In its early days chlorpromazine was thought to damage the liver frequently, but later study showed there had been coincident infective hepatitis; also, the simple test for bile pigments in urine, used to detect occult liver damage, was in fact made positive by metabolites of chlorpromazine alone.

Although many reactions are described in their place elsewhere in this book, it may be helpful to list some reactions that are not always considered.

(a) Rapid rise to high dose

(i) Bizarre movements of tongue, back, or limbs, thought to be attention-seeking ('hysterical') or neurological disease, is dystonia due to neuroleptic (see pp. 82, 84).

(ii) Akinetic mutism or stupor due to neuroleptic raised beyond the Parkinsonian level.

(iii) Ataxia, clumsiness, slurred speech due to high lithium levels.

(b) Rapid withdrawal after long-term treatment

(i) Delirium tremens, from alcohol.
(ii) Epileptic fit, from benzodiazepine or barbiturate.
(iii) Manic attack, from prophylactic lithium.
(iv) Headache, nausea, vomiting, insomnia, from imipramine, or amitriptyline, or a phenothiazine.
(v) Severe Parkinsonism, with rigidity, salivation, urinary retention, from loss of anti-Parkinsonian drug.
(vi) Sudden reduction of high doses may result in confusional state.

(c) Drug interaction

(i) Severe throbbing headache with hypertension and sometimes fever from monoamine oxidase inhibitor with amine drug such as a tricyclic, or ephedrine (in cold cure) (see p. 157).
(ii) Parkinsonism from tricyclic plus lithium.

(d) Obscure

The neuroleptic malignant syndrome, said to be due to high doses of antipsychotics, is described as like Parkinsonism, with raised muscle tone and difficulty in swallowing, raised temperature, raised blood pressure, raised serum creatinine phosphokinase from muscle damage, and variability of pulse and blood pressure and autonomic instability: it is very rare, alarms the doctor, but the patient often recovers if this is waited for. Bromocriptine (15–60 mg daily) has been advocated. Any suspicion of this syndrome should prompt the fullest physical investigation. It is most likely to be a neuroleptic-induced rigidity, possibly with akathisia, and some physical cause of fever.

(e) Unexpected Parkinsonism

Do not forget that haloperidol, even when given for only a short period, can provoke this reaction, which may then continue for up to six months after the drug has been stopped. Also, a drug-free patient who develops a depressive illness may show some signs of Parkinsonism, which will disappear again as the patient recovers. (See also akathisia, p. 82; and tardive dyskinesia, p. 83.)

Reference

KELLAM, A. M. P. (1987) The neuroleptic malignant syndrome, so-called: a survey of the world literature. *British Journal of Psychiatry*, **150**, 752–759.

4 Good prescribing habits

In-patients

The prescription sheet serves three separate but inter-related functions. It is the means of ordering drugs from the pharmacy, it is the instruction sheet for nurses giving patients the drug, and it is also an important part of the patient's record of treatment. On rare occasions it may become a legal document in litigation. Different hospitals have different designs of treatment chart. The following procedures are worth putting into practice.

(a) The patient's surname, first name, hospital number and ward should always be on the prescription sheet. Do not leave it to someone else.
(b) Date the prescription.
(c) Use the proper name of the drug, not its commercial term, unless a particular brand is intended. State the form in which the drug is to be given.
(d) Write, preferably print, in English when the drug is to be given and do not use medical Latin, or abbreviations such as 'b.d.' or 'p.r.n.', which result in error.
(e) Sign the prescription legibly with name as well as initials.
(f) At the same time as you prescribe a drug, write in the case notes what you have prescribed and give a reason, assessing the effects of the previous drug if there was one.
(g) When changing a prescription, date the crossing-out of the previous drug when the new drug is written in.

(h) In long-term patients review medication at least monthly; in acute cases, at least weekly. Check from time to time how the nurses are giving a prescription. For instance, night sedation may be given routinely needlessly, or too early, or daytime sedation may be overused.

Out-patients

The hospital pharmacy may supply drugs for out-patients, usually on a special hospital card; otherwise, drugs for out-patient treatment in the National Health Service (NHS) may be prescribed on Form FP10(HP), pads of which are provided by the hospital. An FP10 form is, in effect, an order to a commercial pharmacist to supply the drugs written on it to the patient whose name appears at the top, in return for payment, part of which is met by the patient and the remainder by the NHS. The FP10 form is also a set of instructions to the chemist about what to write on the label so that patients may know what they are taking, how often to take it and for how long. The FP10 may become a legal document in cases of litigation. Since the FP10 form cannot be a record of treatment unless carbon copies are kept, a note of the prescription should also be made in the patient's case notes, dated and signed. Remember also to observe the following.

With the patient's full name and address at the top, print the proper name of the drug, not its commercial name unless you intend a particular brand to be dispensed. Specify the form in which it is to be dispensed, the frequency with which it is to be taken and the number of tablets, capsules and so on that are to be given to the patient. The dispenser must supply what is written – standard preparation or particular commercial brand.

If you do not wish your patient to know the drug name, delete the letters 'NP' at the top of the prescription form, otherwise the dispenser will write the name of the drug on the container label. Sign and print your name legibly; if there is a mistake the dispenser will be able to contact you.

Explain to patients why the drug is given and tell them, or a responsible relative, how often to take it, what serious side-effects to expect and how to cope with them. Failure to take drugs results in part from poor instruction.

Since the FP10 is in the patient's charge between leaving the out-patient clinic and reaching the dispensing chemist, opportunity for forgery arises. To avoid forgery print the drug name in bold capitals and the quantity in arabic numerals and in words. Leave no free space below the prescription and initial alterations.

Prescriptions ordering controlled drugs (see p. 116) must be handwritten, signed and dated by the prescriber, and always state:

(a) the name and address of the patient
(b) the total quantity of the drug or preparation (and its form), or the number of dose units, in words and figures
(c) the dose.

For drug-dependent patients, daily issue by the chemist, preferably in liquid form, may be a sensible method of rationing the supply and preventing sale of tablets.

Remember, FP10 pads can be stolen and used to forge prescriptions. Lock them up.

5 The cost of treatment

To the National Health Service

The prescriber should have some idea of the price of drugs and, hence, the cost of a course of treatment in the short and long term, so as to make the best use of National Health Service (NHS) money. Even in non-inflationary times, drug prices change. A drug is usually expensive when new and cheaper later, when generic equivalents become available on the expiry of patents. Even so, the more expensive branded preparation may, under certain circumstances, be preferable to the generic product, easier to swallow, more palatable, possess a longer shelf-life after manufacture, or have superior bioavailability.

The approximate cost to the NHS of branded drugs can be obtained from the *Monthly Index of Medical Specialities* (MIMS). MIMS provides, as a guide to prescribing in general practice, a classified list of drugs that may be prescribed or recommended including, for most drugs, the retail price. The *British National Formulary* (BNF) also lists prices, which are based on the average price of dispensing NHS prescriptions. The cost of dispensing a prescription from a retail pharmacy includes the professional fees and overheads, which are not included in MIMS or BNF prices. Hospital pharmacy prices are often much lower than those of retail pharmacists because a local or regional bulk purchasing contract has been arranged with the supplier. The hospital pharmacist will know. To illustrate variable costs, the purchase prices for commonly prescribed psychotropic drugs cited in MIMS (February 1991) are compared with hospital contract prices from one district in Table 1.

TABLE 1

Comparison of drug costs to the NHS: retail (MIMS) prices (excluding VAT) and hospital contract prices (including VAT) (February 1991)

Drugs	*Hospital purchase: £*	*MIMS: £*
Tricyclics: 75 mg a day for 28 days (84 × 25 mg tablets)		
Imipramine	0.52	
'Tofranil'		2.64
Clomipramine	5.63	
'Anafranil'		5.37
Amitriptyline	0.32	
'Lentizol'		3.62
'Tryptizol'		2.13
Newer antidepressants		
Lofepramine: 140 mg daily ('Gamanil', 70 mg tablet) for 28 days	9.51	9.97
Fluoxetine: 20 mg daily ('Prozac', 20 mg tablet) for 28 days	16.10	27.44
Lithium		
1 g a day for 28 days:		
'Camcolit' (250 mg)	1.52	3.25
1600 mg a day for 28 days:		
'Priadel' (400 mg)	1.58	4.16
'Camcolit' (400 mg)	0.76	4.35
Phenothiazines		
400 mg a day for 12 days (48 × 100 mg tablets):		
Chlorpromazine	0.82	
'Largactil'		2.16
Thioridazine	1.39	
'Melleril'		3.84
Syrup:		
Chlorpromazine 25 mg/5 ml (500 ml)	1.21	2.95
Thioridazine 25 mg/5 ml (500 ml)	1.15	3.09
Non-sedative neuroleptics		
Pimozide: 16 mg daily ('Orap' 4 mg tablets) for 28 days	40.52	35.24
Sulpiride: 1200 mg daily ('Dolmatil' 200 mg tablets) for 28 days	27.39	35.28
Trifluoperazine: 20 mg daily ('Stelazine' Spansule 10 mg) for 28 days	3.46	3.01

Syrup takes more time to give than tablets because nursing staff have to measure the dose. Syrup is more expensive than tablets dose for dose, and injections are dearer still.

It is important to know the expensive drugs and prescribe them for a good reason. Anafranil or clomipramine compared with Tryptizol or amitriptyline is an example. But cost can be overemphasised as a factor in clinical decisions. Psychotropic drugs are inexpensive compared with drugs used in general medicine. Concentrate on choosing the right drug without getting distracted by the difference between 3p and 5p a day.

To the patient

All prescriptions written on FP10 forms cost the patient £3.40 (April 1991 price) for each drug dispensed, each time it is dispensed. These charges can be a sizeable financial burden for patients requiring multiple drugs long term, especially if poor as so many patients in continuing care are. However, prescription charges can be mitigated. The NHS has ruled that prescriptions for some medical conditions are exempt from charges. Patients with these conditions do not have to pay charges for their psychotropic drugs. This applies, for instance, to epilepsy, diabetes and thyrotoxicosis. There are other exceptions. The following groups are exempt from prescription charges: children under 16, women over 60, men over 65, pregnant women (Form FW8), women with children under one year (Form FP91/EC91), and people receiving supplementary benefit (income support), family income supplements (family credit), war or service disablement pensions if the treatment is of a condition caused by a disablement.

Prescription charges for patients who have to pay can be reduced with a 'season ticket' which costs £17.60 for four months and £48.50 for 12 months. These are worthwhile for more than six prescribed items or repeats in four months and 15 over a year. 'Season tickets' can be obtained by applying on form FP95/EC95, available from post offices, social security offices, family practitioner committees or retail pharmacists.

Limited prescribing

In April 1986 the Department of Health and Social Security, to reduce the cost of medicines to the NHS, introduced limited prescribing for five categories of medicines. This arose because of arbitrary prescribing of pharmacologically similar preparations of widely varying price. One category deals with tranquillisers and sedatives. As a result, general practitioners can only prescribe, using their generic name, those tranquillisers and sedatives on the approved list. Drugs not prescribable under the NHS are identified in MIMS and the BNF by a symbol. Non-approved drugs can still be prescribed on private prescriptions.

Hospitals are not obliged to follow this restriction and, in many instances, hospital doctors can still prescribe a wider range of psychotropic drugs from their hospital pharmacies than can general practitioners. However, hospital doctors must observe the restrictions if they write prescriptions on FP10 forms for retail pharmacists. Many hospitals have, through consultation between clinicians and pharmacists, developed guidelines for prescribing embodying the principles of the limited list. These district drug formularies, which give information on uses, dosage and costs of selected drugs, have an important role to play in reducing the cost of medicines without sacrificing quality of treatment.

Part II. Notes on management

6 The violent patient

Management

A traditional way of coping with the violence of the mentally ill was by physical restraint: chains, the strait waistcoat, seclusion in the padded cell. Then, in the early 19th century, came the demonstration in England that calm, friendly concern for the individual and simple psychological management made much restraint unnecessary. With the advent of drugs, morphine, hyoscine and the barbiturates became the compellers of peace, in effect by partial anaesthetisation. With modern, more subtle psychotropics which leave consciousness untouched, psychological handling has again become an important component of management. The violent patient presents the most extreme challenge to the psychiatrist of how to combine psychology and pharmacology in effective proportion, a balance needed in the treatment of psychoses and neuroses in general.

In the general hospital ward the psychiatrist may be asked to help not only with the violent but also with cases of lesser disturbance, sometimes involving complex problems of diagnosis or management, and not necessarily to arrange removal of the patient. What the psychiatrist offers is:

(a) a skill in gaining the patient's confidence and a sensitivity to slight pointers in history or behaviour suggesting an organic rather than a psychological origin of symptoms
(b) a standard assessment of mental state, covering all main mental functions

(c) pursuit of a detailed, reliable history, with awareness of the relevance of social and interpersonal factors on the one hand and of the toxic signs of medicines on the other
(d) the ability at times to wait and observe further before drawing conclusions
(e) continuity of care, with only one doctor in charge and keeping medication to the minimum
(f) the use of relatives as well as nurses in management.

Be wary of clever labels and glib interpretations. Be prepared to seek advice from colleagues with more experience.

The accident and emergency centre

Violent and dangerous behaviour is common. Drunks and psychopaths are often quickly recognised and deflected towards the police. Beware of too ready use of 'nuisance' labels and of overlooking mania, schizophrenia, drug-induced psychosis, head injury or a post-epileptic state. Usually, on careful examination, some degree of altered consciousness can be detected here even if no history is available.

Procedure

It is important to have an adequate and defined space for the interview, so that the patient can move about and not feel restricted. It is essential that the doctor appears calm and neutral in manner and can adopt a relaxed, friendly stance. Non-verbal communication matters.

It is impossible to feel confident except with adequate back-up. Do not interview alone but have at least two nurses. Two nurses are not threatening to an excited person, especially if they are seen as carers rather than authority figures. Big numbers of helpers can be threatening.

Be prepared to listen for 30 minutes or more to a patient's stream of complaints. Appear interested in them and do not give meaningless reassurances or unrealistic promises; interpretations and arguments do not help at this stage. It is always possible to move from contentious areas of conversation to less emotionally charged matters.

Whatever the cause, if violent or disturbed behaviour continues and is threatening it may need to be controlled rapidly, and haloperidol, 10–40 mg i.m. or i.v. repeated every two hours until effective, and then changed to 20–40 mg oral dose three times a day, can be used (see p. 177). Alternatively use chlorpromazine (200 mg i.m.) (but not i.v.) two-hourly (but this injection can be painful). The elderly and the less disturbed should have lower doses.

Explain to the patient why and how medication is to be given. Under common law, when actual or potential violence is serious, drugs can be given even without consent. Two or three nurses (either sex, with special training in restraint) can control and inject a patient without causing traumata. The whole procedure, if carefully done, will not later be resented by the patient. Blood can be taken for analysis at the same time, including for glucose and electrolytes.

Rapid, effective control reduces behaviour distressing to patients themselves and results in the possibility of discussion and co-operation in further management.

Drugs used in this way demand close supervision and reassessment every few hours. The search for a firm diagnosis, and the cause of disturbance must be pursued, as this will decide where to place the patient for further treatment (for hypomania, schizophrenia with aggression, delirium tremens, drug-induced psychosis: see under these headings, pp. 53, 73, 87).

Always check that ancillary investigations have been adequate and complete. Blood and urine analysis for drugs is useful to check for toxic levels, for example: phenytoin, tricyclics, barbiturates, aspirin, in overdoses, and where illicit drugs are suspected, amphetamines, codeine, methadone, or morphine. Disturbance apart, patients suffering from toxic effects of drugs (overdose or not) should be treated on medical wards by physicians with expert knowledge. Additional information is available from regional poison units.

7 Mania

Overtalkativeness, overactivity, and overcheerfulness, are the cardinal signs of mania, and increased irritability, distractibility, and a failure of judgement may be obvious too. Irritability leads to verbal and even physical aggression; exasperation with imposed restraints leads to feelings of persecution. Distractibility results in a changeable temper. Lack of judgement may cause irresponsible, impetuous acts which may be criminal or socially unacceptable. A previously well conducted person may start to drink heavily, get involved in fights, become promiscuous. In the milder forms, racing thoughts, without outwardly visible pressure of talk or overactivity may be the only abnormality. Sometimes, those who know the patient can see they are unwell even though talk, mood and activity seem within the norm to strangers.

Manic attacks may develop slowly, taking some days, or rapidly, over a few hours. They may start from a normal state or follow a depressive illness. They may succeed stress, surgery, infection, or childbirth, or follow the use of antidepressants, other drugs or electroconvulsive therapy (ECT). Some are seasonal. This suggests diverse aetiologies leading to a common symptom expression. However, all are managed on the same principles.

Attacks may last a few days, or continue for weeks or months, ending sometimes without treatment. Manic episodes may occur without depression, so called unipolar or bipolar I, or following a major depressive illness with recurring depression dominating the clinical picture, called bipolar II.

Treatment has three aims: managing the patient and the problems created by manic conduct; controlling with drugs the abnormal mental state and behaviour; preventing further attacks.

Managing the patient

Do not argue with the patient – humour him, attempt to establish rapport by discussing the changes he will have noticed, his lack of sleep, his difficulties with family and friends and at work. Use these as the grounds on which he needs your help, possibly with drugs. Maintain gentle, calm, friendly handling, steering him away from extravagant behaviour and indiscretion. Explain to the family that mania is an illness which causes a temporary restlessness, loss of judgement and sense of proportion, from which recovery is expected, so they may be tolerant and forgiving, avoiding challenges. In the first episode the family will need much counselling. Most manic episodes are best treated in hospital, if only to give family and society relief from a trying responsibility. Much skill is needed in achieving this by persuasion. Compulsory admission under the Mental Health Act may be the best method with severe cases, because of refusal to accept treatment or because of the likelihood of poor compliance with drug treatment out of hospital or, indeed, in it.

In hospital, give as much living space as possible; confinement breeds conflict. Two manic patients on a ward can cause chaos. It may be necessary to prevent use of the telephone, to remove cheque books and credit cards, warn the bank, stop car driving and ban business engagements. The patient's demands can be seemingly endless. If you remain firm on limits, understood and agreed by staff, family and associates, patients usually accept them. They may not understand the restrictions but, provided you remain friendly and calm, they may follow them to please you.

Control with drugs

Control of the illness means suppression of overactivity and irritability. Success is measured by reduction of motor restlessness, talkativeness, quarrelsomeness, grandiose ideas and improved sleep. Treatment once begun must be pursued swiftly to success, or the patient will break off and become even more difficult to treat. Because absorption of drugs from tablets is slow or unpredictable, use a syrup or, for the more severe illness, begin with intramuscular or even intravenous injections. It is sometimes possible to persuade the patient to stay in bed for 24 or 48 hours at the start of treatment, out of harm's way, and to minimise the hypotensive effects of drugs. Do not hesitate to use big doses of drugs to get rapid suppression of symptoms. Extrapyramidal side-effects appear only when the mania cools.

In the acute and severely disturbed manic patient the drug of choice is haloperidol or droperidol. Phenothiazines, such as chlorpromazine and thioridazine, will also suppress irritability and produce sedation but are slower acting and less effective than droperidol in leading to normal thinking or in reducing activity. If these drugs fail, even in big doses, or are not available, and the mania is severe and advancing, ECT once daily for two to four days will produce control and ECT twice weekly will do for less severe cases.

The return of the patient's mental state to apparent normality does not allow lessening of clinical vigilance. Within hours or days a swing into a dangerous (suicidal) depressive state may occur. Equally, severe dystonic side-effects may suddenly develop and cause diagnostic confusion.

In acute management, try droperidol or haloperidol 10–40 mg intramuscularly, repeated every two to four hours to achieve control. Usually only two or three doses are needed. As control begins, switch to tablets or syrup (10–20 mg thrice daily), which takes over by degrees from the parenteral drug; the latter can be continued concurrently in reducing dose. In milder forms, start with oral medication (3 mg thrice daily) and increase the dose after 24–48 hours according to response. Results should appear quickly, and the dose be increased or decreased rapidly in the first days of treatment. See the patient frequently, two to three times a day at first, to assess progress, to look for side-effects and the need to change drug or dose. Severe mania is a medical emergency and frequent, careful assessments may be needed for some weeks, until the patient's mood is stable. In the less severe case, try 100 mg of chlorpromazine intramuscularly and repeat, if necessary, every two to three hours. Aim for obvious control and, as soon as there is, start oral doses of 100–300 mg three or four times daily, depending on response.

In milder states, try oral chlorpromazine (50 mg thrice daily) or start lithium carbonate, probably 400 mg four hourly, 8 a.m. to 8 p.m. for four doses, adjusting the dose in the light of the response. With lithium, clinical response will not be achieved until after five or seven days of treatment. Haloperidol, or a phenothiazine, can be safely combined with lithium for those patients who become manic while taking prophylactic lithium.

If haloperidol or lithium fail or cause intolerable side-effects, flupenthixol, trifluoperazine or fluphenazine may be used. Pimozide can be useful. Other potentially effective drugs are carbamazepine, clonazepam and, possibly, sodium valproate. In the elderly patient use smaller doses, or a weaker phenothiazine such as promazine, to lessen the risk of producing a confusional state, urinary incontinence, hypotension and falls.

Prophylaxis

Where attacks of mania or depression occur at intervals of two years or less, and there have been three attacks, prophylaxis with lithium carbonate should be tried. If attacks have been severe and socially disastrous, perhaps only two episodes would justify prophylaxis, but it will rarely be right to start long-term lithium after only one or where recurrences are spaced some years apart.

If lithium fails to prevent recurrences, carbamazepine should be tried. Most bipolar disorders respond to one or other of these drugs, but the few which do not present a formidable clinical and social problem, especially when trying to maintain a patient out of hospital. Here, combining two or more drugs has to be tried. Lithium combined with carbamazepine can be effective when each drug alone has failed. An alternative is to use a neuroleptic instead of lithium. Because poor compliance is so common with mania, haloperidol, droperidol, flupenthixol, fluphenazine, and others, given by depot injection and used in doses similar to those for preventing relapse in schizophrenia, may control manic symptoms or reduce them to a tolerable level.

Resistant bipolar disorders attract polypharmacy. Addition to lithium, one after the other, of a depot neuroleptic, an oral neuroleptic, an anti-Parkinsonian drug, a tricyclic, one benzodiazepine for anxiety and another for insomnia, by psychiatrist and general practitioner striving over a lengthy period of indifferent progress to improve matters, creates a drug fog. Fear of relapse prevents attempts to rationalise overmedication. A sensible course is admission to remove at least some medicines by stages and to review the value of others. If possible, in such cases try to limit medication to a tricyclic, a neuroleptic and lithium.

The few patients who fail drug treatment present serious clinical and social problems. Maintenance out of hospital is threatened by disordered behaviour with crisis after crisis resulting in unplanned admissions. Accommodation with tolerant supervision from family, experienced landlord or group home staff, community nurse involvement, and day hospital attendance which is not demanding on strict adherence to a plan of treatment, may prevent admission to long-stay hospital care. But for a small number, such long-stay institutional care is the better arrangement. Here the patient's overall care can be properly ordered, medication supervised and, if the illness lessens, careful plans made for a further trial outside hospital.

8 Neurotic symptoms

Fears, anxieties, panics, brief bouts of depressive feeling, tension headaches, and nausea are experienced on occasion by nearly everyone, usually in a situation or after an event which justifies such feeling as 'normal'. But in some people symptoms occur where the situation does not seem to call for it, or with greater severity or greater frequency than in the majority. These feelings, which may be termed 'neurotic', may be associated with sweating, rise in pulse rate, palpitations, indigestion, disturbed breathing, urinary frequency or diarrhoea, all well recognised physical correlates of emotions. Apart from their unpleasantness, which leads the patient to seek relief, they are usually associated with some disability in free behaviour. The patient is blocked in some way and cannot undertake certain acts in family, social or sexual relationships or in daily work in spite of a wish to do so. A housewife cannot go outside her front door and becomes very anxious if she tries to do so. One man becomes anxious, possibly impotent, in sexual situations. Another starts to get episodes of sudden panic after two of his workmates have died in quick succession. A third, with promotion at work beyond his abilities, gets incapacitating headaches.

In meeting someone with symptoms of this sort, the first question is diagnosis. Is this patient abnormal, oversensitive in the situation and, if so, in what way? Are these symptoms the tip of the iceberg, and others will be admitted on questioning? How do they change over time? Is this the beginning of a schizophrenic illness or an episode of depressive illness in which depressive mood has not yet appeared but other signs of biological depression are there: early-waking insomnia, loss of appetite, impaired concentration, lack of energy? Anyone over 40 in whom 'neurotic' symptoms are appearing for the first time is probably suffering either from an attack of depressive illness or from some hidden organic disease, possibly a pre-senile dementia, temporal lobe epilepsy or a carcinoma.

Or are we dealing with a person of abnormal personality who, through a sort of emotional colour blindness, keeps running into unexpected social and emotional difficulties not experienced by the majority and reacting in an upset, angry or depressed way? Occasionally, this seems to be constitutional in origin. In other cases, unusual earlier experiences and mistaken learning seem to exert a powerful influence in the present. The patient cannot run away from some current experience nor face it and act, but remains in inner conflict over what to do. These people may be classified as neurotic or as suffering from a personality disorder.

If one identifies what situation provokes the anxiety or other symptoms, one can help the patient to avoid it without shame or, better, it may be possible to change it for him so that it no longer challenges and upsets. But one can also lessen the patient's degree of self-concern, which will have built up on top of the original difficulties. Giving patients plenty of interview time suggests the therapist values them and encourages them to feel better about themselves. They learn that they are not alone, that others have similar troubles, that one can talk openly about them and not be criticised or condemned. No guilt or shame attaches to them. They also begin to learn to understand their troubles, not to interpret symptoms as always indicators of physical illness but sometimes of internal emotion or unhelpful reactions to stresses which have become established over the years. They see factors at work which they previously ignored or of which they were unaware. The human mind hungers for explanation and patients may need to be given this to explain their own hypersensitivity in terms of a present illness, past mis-education or family dynamics. Patients also appreciate an account of the disturbed physiology which leads to such distressing somatic symptoms.

Feeling that the therapist understands a patient's case raises hope for the future. Hope may lessen symptoms, and milder or less frequent symptoms may allow spontaneous improvement to follow as illness is not reinforced by more attacks. In some cases, a single hour with the therapist can be enough to start recovery. Suppression of symptoms with a drug is also very helpful. It brings the patient relief, it displays the therapist's power to help, it stops reinforcement of the illness. Except in those who are using illness to protect themselves from something they want to avoid, removal of symptoms does not result in new complaints but in general benefit.

Psychotherapy of a more advanced kind, whether analytical or behavioural, individual or group or family, is an attempt to re-educate the patient, and sometimes close family too, so that earlier and partly buried misconceptions cease to inhibit or to create conflict. Cognitive therapy can prove very effective, selection depending on the patient's personality, co-operation and intelligence. These methods are time consuming and not suitable for everyone; fortunately a good deal can be done without them, especially if drugs are used where they can help, and not withheld on some theoretical or moral ground. There is no law that psychological problems can only be treated by psychology, or that only the patient's own efforts are to be valid. The aim must be to spare suffering and increase the freedom to act as patients wish within the law. Obviously, where neurotic symptoms are part of depressive illness or schizophrenia or organic disease, medication of the main illness will be important. But, where they are localised in a small maladaptive segment of the patient's total behaviour, with very limited symptoms, medication plays a smaller and usually short-term role. Planning a treatment, and expectations from it, must be appropriate to the pattern of illness and distinction made between acute, acute becoming chronic and the very chronic picture.

Situational anxiety

Someone becoming anxious and panicky before an important job interview, a student with worry and insomnia before an examination, a patient awaiting the dentist or the first session of electroconvulsive therapy, someone distraught after an acute life crisis (death of child, unexpected departure of spouse) are examples of acute trouble, where a hypnotic or a daytime sedative, in either case in single dose, may be helpful. The hypnotic must be effective, without hangover, and may need to be repeated for two or three nights at most. The sedative is taken half to one hour before the feared experience, and it is very advisable to try it out beforehand to get the dose and timing right, so that it is neither too strong nor too weak at the time its support is wanted. The person who becomes upset at having to eat in a public restaurant, or to be a passenger in an aeroplane, can be helped in the same way, although some psychological treatment may be more curative in the long-run for them. Short-acting benzodiazepines, such as temazepam (10 mg) or triazolam (0.125 mg) (see section on these drugs, pp. 188–194), or sodium amylobarbitone (200–400 mg) or thioridazine or chlorpromazine (50–100 mg by mouth) are three types of hypnotic which apply. Although the first two types are potentially addictive, such very short use is harmless. Bear in mind, though, that stopping a hypnotic often means a poor night or more following, until normality is reasserted. For daytime use, diazepam (2 or 5 or even 10 mg) once only an hour beforehand may be right, and can be repeated only before later stressful events of the same character. Oxazepam (10 mg or 15 mg) is another alternative, as is chlorpromazine (10–25 mg) or fluanxol (0.5 mg).

Abnormal reactions to situations can be the result of some frightening incident in the past which may have been forgotten. Abreaction (see under Appendix 2, p. 229) is sometimes helpful in disclosing this. Relaxed by an intravenous drug, the patient (in a more suggestible condition) can be induced to talk frankly about relevant emotional experiences and to recall exceptionally potent events. Talking about them into full consciousness may remove their force. Hysterical amnesia and paralysis may be relieved in this way.

Chronic anxiety and fears

Some patients develop free-floating anxiety, not obviously related to any situations, though it often waxes and wanes over periods of weeks. It may be present on and off at least from adolescence, or it may start in adult life after some minor incident and then continue for a long period. It can be made worse by an environment which cannot be evaded: excessive noise, crowded children in a cramped home, or an unpleasant office where work must go on. Relaxation can be taught, attempts made to clarify the historical origins of the disturbance and disability, and the principles of cognitive or behaviour therapy applied. But it may be humane, or essential, to suppress the symptoms if the patient is to continue at work; psychological methods may fail and other treatment demanded. Amitriptyline or thioridazine (10 mg three times a day of either) may be tried first.

Benzodiazepines may be needed in severe anxiety. Because of their liability to produce dependence, with the risk of escalating dose and the impossibility of withdrawal without producing unpleasant symptoms, they should only be prescribed for limited periods (maximum one month) in the lowest workable dose, and on a time schedule which recognises that some of these drugs are metabolised to longer-acting forms. Thus, diazepam has a major effect over four hours, but a chronic effect due to its metabolites comes later and this effect may build up slowly, day by day, so that less drug is needed; for example, give 5 mg diazepam three times a day and then perhaps 2 mg three times a day, although it is best not to choose a rigid schedule of this sort but tailor one to the patient's life. Oxazepam is not metabolised in this way and may, therefore, be preferable.

Where attacks of panic are predominant, a tricyclic antidepressant, imipramine or amitriptyline, starting in low doses (25 mg twice daily) and working up to those used for depression (150 mg a day) may work well. In severe cases neuroleptics, orally or even by depot injection, may be very helpful. Where bodily symptoms of sweating, palpitations, etc., are important, propranolol (30–60 mg daily) may lessen anxiety, although it directly touches the physical rather than the mental symptoms. Phenelzine (15–90 mg daily) also has a place, particularly if generalised phobic symptoms dominate the picture. In obsessive–compulsive states, clomipramine is the most effective but other tricyclics up to 300 mg daily, or chlorpromazine (300 mg daily), can be tried. In a few cases nothing seems to work except amylobarbitone in regular doses over a long period. This illustrates one of the conflicts of medicine. The drug has a high risk of inducing dependence; on the other hand it may be the only way which enables a patient to go to work and support a family. It is less difficult treating the suffering of a man of 66, where dependence is a less serious matter than, say, at 46. In many cases, dependence does not mean dose escalation or a change towards harder drugs, and therefore may be less worrying. Taking all the individual factors into account and trying to come to a fair and balanced decision for that individual seems the only approach, rather than absolute rules.

Chronic illness implies regular reassessment from time to time, measuring relief against target symptoms, and a willingness to re-think treatment. It may need to be altered as people change. Be alert to a sudden symptom change, indicating a depressive illness with risk of suicide in one previously with chronic neurotic disability only. Always have a systematic plan of follow-up.

9 Depressive illness

Depression is the name of a feeling and is usually but not always accompanied by a sad face, tears, or complaints of gloom and pessimism. The doctor is only called in when the feeling seems inappropriate in strength, duration, or occasion. To feel depressed for a few hours now and then is normal, but to be depressed for days, weeks or months on end is quite another matter. This inappropriate depression may be a primary part of the symptom complex of a depressive illness, or a secondary consequence of some other illness or disability. Discrimination between these possibilities affects the treatment.

The psychiatrist judges the inappropriateness of depressed mood by comparing the patient's feeling and behaviour with that of others, and more especially with that of people who resemble the patient in sex, race, and social background. If you know the patient or have the advice of someone who does, you may decide the feeling and behaviour are inappropriate for that patient, because the patient is different from his/her individual norm, even though the difference does not fall outside the normal range for such people. Some patients can recognise this finer degree of inappropriateness in themselves.

The more intense the depression, the more likely it is to be associated with other symptoms here termed the 'biological response' – sleep disturbance, loss of appetite, loss of weight, loss of libido, loss of drive, fatigue, loss of interests, increased anxieties and impaired concentration. The wish to sleep for ever, for life to come to an end, even the idea of ending life may be there also and must be asked about. The presence and severity of these symptoms, not necessarily all of them, in association with depressive feeling is a measure of the patient's psychobiological response, whether to external emotional stresses, or to internal bodily disturbances.

The more pronounced the biological response the more likely it is that physical methods of treatment will be helpful.

Some patients do not admit to depressed feelings. They may, however, be preoccupied with their physical and mental health. Their complaints may be of pains, headache, loss of all interest, inexplicable anxiety, fear of serious illness, or compulsive thoughts. Only when directly asked do they admit to psychobiological symptoms. These patients are examples of masked depression, to be treated with antidepressants or electroconvulsive therapy (ECT) like other depressive illnesses. Such patients may be first referred by their general practitioners to physicians and surgeons, who must be aware that depressions can masquerade as other illnesses.

Some patients are preoccupied by past failures. Depression sometimes seems reactive to life situations, especially loss events – loss of loved ones, loss of self-esteem through failures in work, the declining powers of middle age, sudden misfortunes, sexual disappointments. At times depression seems inexplicable. But life stresses, whether present or absent, are irrelevant in deciding to use ECT or psychotropic drugs. It is not the supposed stress but the patient's biological responses to it which matter in choosing the treatment. Ignore presumed causes and concentrate on the pattern of symptoms in deciding on drug management of the case. Always bear in mind the risk of suicide (see Appendix 3).

Recognition of the circumstances that provoke depressive illness may however indicate the need for emotional re-education when the acute phase of the illness is over, with psychotherapy, or planned social readjustment. These approaches are used more to strengthen the patient against future illness than to relieve the present one. General psychological nursing of the patient in hospital may reduce the severity of depressive symptoms, but usually this effect is temporary. If there is no sustained improvement after ten days, it may be dangerous not to proceed with physical methods of treatment.

Secondary depressions

People of less ability than their social manner indicates may find themselves in jobs or situations beyond their capacity and may become depressed by failure. People of abnormal personality get into troubles that others avoid, and may become depressed by the consequences. People whose memories and intellectual capacities fail early, for instance in organic dementia before 60, may present with depression as their abilities diminish. Depression can be an important symptom in conditions associated with brain damage, head injury, epilepsy, Parkinsonism, multiple sclerosis, with rheumatoid arthritis and other chronic disabilities. Cancer, some endocrine disorders, vitamin deficiencies, and viral infections also seem to be associated with depression. Some drugs predispose to depression; others, if stopped after long use, may result in depression. Secondary depressions may therefore have psychological or physiological causes, and sometimes both. In such cases both the primary condition and the depression itself may need to be treated.

Many attempts have been made to subdivide depressive illness into groups with distinctive treatments. Some classifications used stages of life (e.g. involutional melancholia, puerperal depression), others the timing of recurrences (e.g. seasonal depression, rapid cyclers, unipolar and bipolar); yet others used biochemical tests suggesting distinct serotonergic or noradrenergic types. None of this has proved of use in everyday practice.

Early action

Much of what is said in this section may apply also to the care of acute situational depression, or other acute secondary depressions without the symptoms of biological response.

The first step is to ensure a good night's sleep, using 10–50 mg temazepam, 5–20 mg nitrazepam, 50–150 mg chlorpromazine or thioridazine in one dose, or amitriptyline in the same dose range. Size of dose depends on weight, age, physical health, previous experience of the drug. It is better to achieve excessive sleep the first night and then reduce the dose, than to start with doses of small effect and then cautiously advance night by night. Control should be swift. Formerly barbiturates were much used because they are effective, but barbiturates produce hangovers, stimulate drug metabolism so that other drugs become less effective, and carry risks of suicide or drug dependence. They must, therefore, only be used when other drugs are known to be ineffective, and then with thought and caution.

If there is anxiety or restlessness, day sedatives from once daily to four-hourly in severe cases will help in the short term. Here the dosage must be more cautious because of the risk of drowsiness, confusion and falling: single doses of diazepam (2–10 mg), oxazepam (10–30 mg), chlorpromazine (50 mg), thioridazine (50 mg), flupenthixol (0.5–1.5 mg) or amitriptyline (10–20 mg) may assist. If barbiturates have to be used for extreme agitation give amylobarbitone (50–200 mg). Relief of distress by day, like improvement of sleep by night, may start a general lifting of the depression and the drug may not be needed long in less severe cases.

The depressed person often feels alone. Mustering the concern of relatives and friends may be helpful. A temporary change of environment, such as staying with a friend, may bring some relief. Admission to hospital may relieve environmental anxieties and obligations but should not be rushed into. Admission may well be correct where there is a serious risk of suicide or of danger to others, or of antisocial behaviour, or where there is a particularly unhelpful environment. On occasion, compulsory admission will be life-saving. However, the depressed person who is still working may not need to stop work, or have everyday social links and responsibilities taken away. Separation of mother and baby is probably bad for both (most hospitals now have mother and baby units). Hospital admission for a mental illness can have stigmatising consequences, prejudicing the patient's future employment, emigration, or child adoption. The person with an acute depressive reaction, seemingly precipitated by some life event, and the mildly depressed person, particularly if obsessional, or where anxious or hypochondriacal symptoms are prominent, may improve in a few days and stay well simply with refreshing sleep and some daytime sedation. If not, or the improvement is temporary, lasting say only 7–14 days, then specific treatment is indicated.

Specific treatment

The most effective treatment is ECT because of its speed of response and rate of success compared with drugs. ECT is safe, suitable for the pregnant, the over-80s, those with healed coronary infarcts and other physical illnesses. Advice on technique, how many treatments to give, how to judge improvement, is given in Appendix 2. Although ECT is so effective, a tricyclic antidepressant drug such as imipramine, amitriptyline or dothiepin should be tried first, especially in out-patients. The greater sureness and speed of ECT is valuable where, for example, the depression is severe, or there is serious risk of suicide, or if it is urgent for someone to return to work or to young children.

The antidepressant action of tricyclic drugs may take up to 10 days or more to begin. Give 25 mg thrice daily for two days, then 50 mg thrice daily for 12 days. If there is no sign of improvement at this stage, and side-effects insignificant, the dose can be increased to 75 mg and occasionally even to 100 mg three times daily. Be guided by the severity of side-effects in limiting dosage. In milder cases 100 mg daily may suffice. Dothiepin is less potent than amitriptyline and a daily dose of less than 100 mg will have only a placebo effect. Imipramine and, even more, amitriptyline have a sedative action and doses of 50–100 mg at night usually make a hypnotic unnecessary. To control restlessness or anxiety a benzodiazepine or a phenothiazine can be added, in the doses quoted above (p. 65), and used to control distress for only a limited period. Patients metabolise and destroy drugs at varying rates, which is why different people require different doses.

Side-effects are worse in the first days of treatment, or just after each dose increase. The patient who has had the purpose and side-effects of the drug explained is more likely to tolerate a dry mouth and other side-effects without asking for the treatment to be changed. If the sedative effect is excessive, or postural hypotension a problem, changing to a less sedative tricyclic such as nortriptyline may produce less severe side-effects. Laboratory measurement of plasma levels of antidepressant is occasionally helpful in adjusting dosage to avoid severe side-effects or poor therapeutic response. Related, newer, drugs such as lofepramine, mianserin and trazodone are used in the individual patient to avoid severe anticholinergic or possible cardiac effects.

The whole of a day's dose can be taken on one occasion if side-effects do not prevent it: the customary ritual thrice daily has no other advantage because tricyclics have long half-lives. In fact, taking a large dose at night when the patient is lying down minimises the hypotensive and other side-effects: the patient is asleep when he might be experiencing them. A single daily dose also aids compliance. Treatment must be continued after symptoms have gone, probably for several months. After four weeks of being well the dose may be reduced by stages, one or two weeks at each level, the return of symptoms being looked for. Do not reduce the dose just as the patient leaves hospital, or resumes his job, or is exposed to special stress. Choose a socially stable and quiet time. Too early cesssation of drugs may result in an avoidable relapse, discouraging to the patient, the family and the employer.

If amitriptyline, imipramine or dothiepin in doses of up to 300 mg a day for a month do not work, changing to another tricyclic is not likely to improve matters. Adding lithium carbonate to the tricyclic may produce an improvement in a few days. Otherwise a complete change of medication is indicated, or ECT used. ECT is compatible with tricyclic treatment and, where tricyclics alone have failed, ECT may succeed. Their combined use can produce the best result for severe depressions.

Alternative treatment

Where tricyclics fail, monoamine oxidase inhibitor (MAOI) drugs may succeed, either alone or, exceptionally, combined with tricyclics. These drugs are quite different from tricyclics in mode of action and their value less well defined. They also carry special dangers and distinct dietary disadvantages. They may be effective for 'atypical depressions', in which depressive feeling coexists with lack of energy, easy fatigue, hypochondriacal complaints and phobic anxieties, and insomnia, if present, is not of the early-waking type, depressive delusions absent, concentration is unimpaired and weight loss and other bodily symptoms lacking.

Monoamine oxidase inhibitors are slower to act on mood than are tricyclics but occasionally produce impressive results in typical as well as atypical cases, especially those with pronounced anxiety. Phenelzine is the most commonly prescribed. Continue for four weeks and up to dosage of 90 mg daily before deciding that treatment has failed. If successful, phenelzine should be continued for some weeks after the disappearance of symptoms and then gradually discontinued, reducing the dose by 15 mg each week. Tranylcypromine and isocarboxazid are useful alternatives. The effect of MAOI drugs continues for up to four weeks after the patient has stopped taking them, the time required to synthesise fresh enzyme to replace that inactivated by the drug.

When MAOIs and tricyclics separately have failed, an MAOI and a tricyclic in combination may work. The drugs may be started together, the MAOI in the morning and the tricyclic in the evening to make best use of any sedative effect, or the tricyclic may be started first (p. 156). Phenelzine and amitriptyline are commonly used. High blood pressure and other combination side-effects must be looked for. The treatment is therefore best started in hospital, where good observation is possible. Otherwise, the patient should be seen every second or third day as an out-patient. The doses of tricyclic drug and MAOI may be increased, depending on symptom response and side-effects, in small increments to the maximum dose levels of each, as if used on its own.

Tranylcypromine in such combination is particularly associated with side-effects of hypotensive faints, headache and insomnia.

L-tryptophan (3–6 g daily) either alone or combined with a tricyclic or an MAOI was believed to be useful in depressive illness resistant to these two drugs used alone. Tryptophan has now been withdrawn because it may be responsible for the eosinophilia–myalgia syndrome.

Treatment failure

Physical treatments are not always effective. For the depressed patient who remains ill, try to identify the area of failure. Was the right dose prescribed? Did the patient take the drug as instructed? Did the side-effects prevent a high enough dose being achieved? If so, try a different drug of the same family or a slower build-up to a bigger dose. Were therapeutic levels ever achieved? Lack of side-effects may be a pointer to failure here. The effects of phenytoin, carbamazepine and other drugs concurrently taken may decrease drug levels. Laboratory measurements help to decide if plasma levels are within the therapeutic range. If levels are too low, try just exceeding the recommended upper dose limit; if too high a lower dose may work.

Has the symptom pattern changed, even though recovery is incomplete? For example, the treatment may have caused a switch from depression to hypomania, or may have abolished the biological symptoms of a depressive illness but with the patient retaining the sick role and exhibiting anxiety symptoms, or depressive symptoms may have cleared, uncovering an unsuspected dementia with consequent inadequacies of function.

Failure of treatment should lead to review of the diagnosis. Is there an unrecognised medical illness? Is there a neurosis or personality disorder as well as depression?

A planned programme of drugs and ECT, with the treatment and response recorded, enables a confident conclusion about the effectiveness or otherwise of each, in defined dose and circumstance. The record is invaluable because the failed treatments need not then be tried again in later episodes, avoiding unneeded suffering and delay.

Most depressive illnesses recover spontaneously, even after years. When depression is not too distressing or handicapping, waiting is probably the best course. But can the patient wait? Is the distress too severe or the risk of suicide too great? Is there too little waiting time because of age or incurable physical illness? Leucotomy, now rarely used, may provide relief in these less common circumstances.

Even the most effective drug treatment does not usually restore to full health immediately. A return to complete personal and social competence may take many months after removal of the most distressing and disabling symptoms. Sometimes, reversion to pre-illness health is never achieved, leaving a deficit which can last indefinitely. Attempts to treat the deficit may cause more harm than good.

Preventing further illness

Antidepressant drugs begin by suppressing symptoms rather than abolishing the underlying malfunction. If the drugs are stopped as soon as the patient has lost all symptoms, relapse is likely. Therefore continue the drug treatment for, say, a further three months but with reducing dosage to allow time for the illness to resolve, whether by natural remission or from drug action.

One depressive illness, or one manic attack, indicates a risk of further attack. There may be years of health before the illness recurs, or only a few months. A third episode may follow the second after a shorter time, and a fourth come sooner still. What can be done to prevent attacks or reduce their severity? Prophylaxis by physical treatment is only appropriate where the illness recurs frequently (say within three years or less).

Although so good at ending depressive illness, ECT is useless for prophylaxis. The three agents of proven value are tricyclic antidepressants, lithium and, less certainly, carbamazepine. Amitriptyline, dothiepin, nortriptyline, imipramine and probably other tricyclics prevent the recurrence of depression. They should be used in the same dose found effective for the patient's episode of acute depression. Because they appear to predispose to mania, tricyclics should not be used for prophylaxis of bipolar disorder. Lithium is the best established prophylactic agent against recurrent depression (see also its use in recurrent hypomania, p. 136). A steadily maintained plasma level of 0.5–0.7 mmol/l of lithium is preventative of both depressive and manic attacks. If lithium also fails, carbamazepine can be substituted. Carbamazepine appears to be superior to lithium in rapid-cycling bipolar illness. Tentative evidence suggests that carbamazepine and lithium together may be effective when either alone is not. When an illness is periodically recurrent, perhaps seasonal, to start or stop antimanic and antidepressant drugs in tune with its rhythm may only emphasise it. A long-term plan is better.

Other measures have a place in prophylaxis besides drugs. Psychotherapy and environmental adjustment through social work can be most helpful, especially when directed at events or circumstances that appeared to have developed just before the onset of the illness.

10 Schizophrenia

Patients with schizophrenia may show a great variety of behavioural and subjective symptoms and signs. A given individual may only suffer a selection of them, and symptoms may be different at different times in the course of a single illness. Thus there may be inactivity and withdrawal from others and the environment in general, restlessness and emotional fluctuations to extremes of panic or suspicion, inappropriate laughter or sadness, the experience of auditory and tactile hallucinations, the expression of delusional ideas, or thinking may clearly be derailed.

Neuroleptic drugs are very useful in the suppression of such active symptoms and signs, but they are not curative (or specifically antischizophrenic), and form only a part of the modern management of the illness. They are important in four circumstances:

(a) emergency control of acute disturbances
(b) suppression of many of the symptoms in the acute illness
(c) suppression of exacerbation in the chronically ill
(d) prevention of recurrence of illness in those who have largely recovered.

In long-term care (c and d above) it becomes very evident that there is a whole range of abnormal behaviour unaffected by drugs – emotional flatness and indifference, inertia and anergy, and poverty of interests and responsiveness. Some of these – a defect state – may be present after recovery from an acute illness, or form the major disability in a chronically ill patient, and these defects can be responsible for an otherwise normal-seeming person proving unable to work or maintain social relationships.

A clinical interview lasting 5 to 50 minutes may not reveal either active symptoms or even more the negative defect state. Therefore independent accounts from those who see the patient every day (family, friends, neighbours, work-mates) indicating how he/she has been behaving in different situations may be essential to a good assessment. It also points to the need to advise and help the family to cope with the patient at home. Sufferers can hide symptoms either deliberately, for example when paranoid, or from indifference and poor concentration in replying to questions. Conversely, certain stress situations, such as fatigue, criticism, presumed antagonisms, or strange experiences, evoke fears of inability to cope with the world and an acute exacerbation of positive symptoms results. Stresses on an individual may vary from day to day or hour to hour but, because of their illness, schizophrenic people have an abnormal sensitivity to such events which render them more vulnerable. Psychotropic drugs appear to lessen this sensitivity.

The disturbed patient

Aggressive or disturbed behaviour is now the usual reason for admitting patients with schizophrenia to hospital. Anaesthetisation with barbiturates or morphine and hyoscine used to be all that was possible. With modern drugs, targets for suppression are hostility and dangerous behaviour, irritability and restlessness, but without reducing consciousness. The drugs used in early treatment are given for disturbance in larger doses, as syrup or by intramuscular, occasionally even by intravenous, injection. Chlorpromazine (100–200 mg), droperidol or haloperidol (10–30 mg), all given orally or intramuscularly, every two to four hours, initially, should achieve rapid control within one or two days, and then give three to four times daily. In a crisis, intravenous haloperidol (10–30 mg) can be used. By the third or fourth day, as the patient improves, regular oral medication, syrup or tablets, should suffice. The change-over to oral doses requires care. A common error is to start off well and then lose control again through inadequate dosage. Start the oral drug while continuing but gradually lessening the injected doses and frequency. Careful monitoring of change is required for the ensuing two to three weeks. After absorbing large quantities of drug during an acute phase, patients may suddenly develop marked side-effects, such as drowsiness or acute dystonic reactions. The latter can be mistaken for symptoms of the illness. Anti-Parkinsonian drugs may be needed, at times by injection, and antipsychotic drugs reduced.

Early treatment

This may be in hospital or at home. Patients often improve considerably once away from the stresses of home and ordinary life, particularly if the hospital offers a simple, calm routine. Through their illness they may suffer doubts and confusions about themselves, the world, and their relation to others; emotional relations with mother and father may be particularly upsetting. A clear structure for a basic daily pattern of activities, including getting up, washing, shaving, using make-up and other self-care, meals and manageable tasks, either domestic or occupational therapy, helps them to return to reality and feel more effective. Permissiveness, on the contrary, may engender further confusion.

One or two nurses must make a special effort to befriend the patient; the establishment of a relationship even though, at times, seemingly tenuous, superficial or difficult is always therapeutic provided it does not become too close. This means that the ward staff must have a constancy from day to day and week to week and not be subject to frequent posting, and they must be correctly identifiable by patients.

The building of confidence allows the patient to enter positively into the life of the ward and to co-operate with treatment, largely free of attacks of distress or violence. These objectives apply also to those treated in a day hospital or as out-patients but efforts may be needed to persuade regular attendance. Supervision, by regular visiting from a community nurse, is an invaluable part of treatment maintenance and allows for family and associates to report progress or setbacks.

Initial assessment of the patient means: (a) making sure that the illness falls in the schizophrenic group and is not an acute brain syndrome or an atypical manic–depressive disorder, for which the treatment and prognosis are different; (b) identifying symptoms – delusions, hallucinations, passivity feelings, poor concentration, paranoid thinking – which can be targets of attack by drug, the subsequent decline of symptoms serving as a guide to drug dosage; (c) judging whether immediate prognosis is good, from the acuteness of onset, the precipitating stresses including the taking of illicit drugs (especially stimulants), and the presence of affective and other positive symptoms; (d) identifying family or social stresses which may assist or retard recovery.

If the patient is not distressed, give a non-sedative neuroleptic such as trifluoperazine (10 mg twice daily), sulpiride (400 mg twice daily) or pimozide (8 mg twice daily) for one or two weeks, by which time symptoms should have lessened. If not, raise the dose gradually (with sulpiride up to 2400 mg daily) and review weekly. In the distressed patient, more sedative phenothiazines or butyrophenones are usually used. Start with chlorpromazine or thioridazine (100 mg thrice daily) again for one or two weeks, and then review. With experience, one learns to gauge from the severity of illness the dosage that will probably be required and to increase it, by steps, perhaps even to 800 mg chlorpromazine or 20 mg fluphenazine, the most potent per weight in this series of drugs. Start with lower doses and build up gradually because side-effects, especially dystonic reactions, become severe if time for adaptation is not allowed. Parkinsonism is often induced at the higher levels and must be treated with anti-Parkinsonian drugs if it appears.

Some patients unwilling to take tablets are prepared to drink syrup, which is more quickly and regularly absorbed, and cannot secretly be got rid of by a paranoid patient. To start with, all the day's dose can be given at night as 'sleeping medicine', which some patients will accept while refusing daytime drugs. More rarely, those who refuse tablets or syrup will be prepared to have intramuscular injections. With tablets by mouth one can never be sure the patient is taking them and this may be a reason for phenothiazines seeming to fail. Even if the patient has not expressed concern, it is important to inquire after side-effects, without alarming the patient.

Failure to treat schizophrenia successfully with phenothiazines commonly arises because: (a) the patient is not getting the drug; (b) the doctor has been overcautious and not prescribed big enough doses; (c) the doctor has not waited long enough (at least a week) for improvement; (d) the doctor is making a global assessment only of behavioural improvement instead of watching for the decline of individual symptoms (hallucinations becoming infrequent and less forceful, concentration improving, restlessness declining). Even if there is no global improvement, the drugs may have produced a change in the symptom pattern, which shows they are doing something and can perhaps be used to better effect in larger doses or on a different schedule or by a different route. Some patients who do poorly with phenothiazines will do better with butyrophenones. Start with, for example, 3 mg haloperidol thrice daily and increase dosage in steps to 60 mg daily, in divided doses, before deciding it is ineffective; or pimozide (8 mg or more, in steps up to 20 mg) can be used. Anti-Parkinsonian drugs may be required but only in a proportion of patients.

Those patients who fail to lose their active symptoms on drugs alone may do better if given a course of electroconvulsive therapy (ECT) while the drug is continued. But defect-state disabilities are *not* helped by ECT. Do not go beyond a maximum of five treatments unless improvement is clearly occurring after each treatment but do not be put off if the first two ECT sessions seem to do nothing. ECT by itself usually has only a temporary (48-hour) suppressant effect on symptoms, except in the case of acute catatonia and acute thought disorder. Combined with phenothiazines, the effects can be lasting. Note that combination of lithium with a neuroleptic may also improve symptom suppression.

Early improvement is shown by modification of symptoms. Later assessment is by observing the patient's abilities to mix with others, to concentrate and to make realistic decisions, and his capacity to undertake work and persist at it. The observations of nurses and relatives are essential here. Do not increase doses further when these improvements appear.

Once improvement is marked, the daily drug dose should be cautiously reduced by steps every two to three weeks, watching for the return of symptoms as a sign to reduce the dose no further. Appearance of a confusional state, or of a compulsive restlessness or internal feeling of unrest (akathisia), or of drowsiness by day, are also indications to reduce drug intake. Drugs may be stopped after a first episode of illness if the patient remains well for three months and where the prognosis is thought to be good. Observe carefully over the next 12 weeks for the return of symptoms.

Remember, however, that a schizophrenic illness can have a disastrous effect on the course of a person's life, for instance the prospects of a career and marriage. Choose the time for managing without drugs with great care so that if, by ill chance, a relapse does occur, it will not fall at a critically upsetting time for the patient. For example, a student who has a schizophrenic breakdown in the final year at college should be carried through examinations and well into a first job before considering drug withdrawal.

Where drugs even in high doses for a maximum of two months seem to make little difference to the patient's illness, they should be withdrawn step-wise over a week or so. Sudden cessation may result in vomiting and malaise.

With lessening in-patient hospital facilities, more patients are managed in the community, perhaps attending as day patients or being closely monitored as out-patients by community psychiatric nurses. Counselling of the family to manage home relationships is then essential. But the principles of drug treatment remain the same. Then it is particularly important for the patient to be reviewed regularly, for example weekly at first, monthly later, and for someone who lives with the patient to be regularly asked about him or her.

Long-term management and prevention of relapse

Some schizophrenics become completely well. The patient who has had a first schizophrenic illness of short duration, who is symptom-free and has been off all drugs for 12 weeks in the community, can be discharged from psychiatric observation. Others continue to require drugs to suppress their hallucinatory experiences or their morbid suspicion of people around them, or may develop a depressive illness requiring antidepressant drugs. In others, psychotic experiences remit but disabling residual symptoms remain against which drugs have little effect.

These residual symptoms are of three kinds. Most common is a lack of energy, a lack of drive and inability to think coherently: although expressing the best intentions and seemingly fit, the patient in the extreme case is quite unable to work, and in many less extreme cases cannot manage a day's work at normal speed. Second is a lack of feeling, particularly an indifference to or unawareness of the feelings of others: the graces of social behaviour are dropped. Third is a preoccupation with eccentric ideas, which may force the patient, and perhaps family, to live in a restricted or unusual way.

Most patients who continue on drugs because they would be worse without them will be living out of hospital, 'in the community', some at work, leading some semblance of a normal life. Some will be symptom-free, others will have some symptoms. It may need good judgement to decide whether these symptoms are drug side-effects or residual disease effects. Slowness in movement and mental dulling may result from incomplete suppression of Parkinsonian symptoms, drowsiness and inattention to excessive phenothiazine, or to the disease process.

During long-term drug treatment, assess from time to time how drugs are helping the patient. Look back over the history, the early symptoms before treatment started, the chronic course of management. Pay particular attention to anti-Parkinsonian drugs which may no longer be necessary, perhaps having been started in other circumstances. Minor tranquillisers or antidepressants, useful at an earlier treatment stage, may not be required. The antipsychotic drug, itself the mainstay of the drug regime, may have become inappropriate in dose or schedule. Trying out changes of the drug regime, while looking for behavioural and symptom change either good or bad in the patient, may be needed to demonstrate what the regime is actually doing. Too many patients are found continuing on a multiplicity of drugs, for example an oral phenothiazine as well as a depot, benzodiazepine and anti-Parkinsonian drugs, perhaps an antidepressant as well, sometimes for years. Medication should not become a standard routine but be revised regularly and cut down on a rational basis. Reduce slowly and be aware what the initial key symptoms of relapse are likely to be in each individual (see p. 174).

It is important to remember that apathy and anergy are often signs of a schizophrenic illness itself and not a consequence of institutionalisation or of drugs; nor will drugs affect these signs favourably.

Schizophrenics may suffer attacks of depressive illness, which can be treated with tricyclic drugs like other depressions. But sometimes depressive symptoms appear as the antipsychotic drug is reduced, and will disappear again as the drug is increased without other treatment.

Taking tablets several times a day without fail can be difficult. Tablets which only need to be taken once a day, such as pimozide, are easier but better still are the long-acting depot injections of phenothiazine derivatives (fluphenazine decanoate) or thioxanthenes (e.g. flupenthixol decanoate) or butyrophenones (haloperidol decanoate). A single painless intramuscular injection, perhaps once a month though sometimes more often, may suffice as maintenance treatment. Such long-term treatment not only suppresses symptoms but prevents future relapse. Injections are started and then the oral medication withdrawn in stages. However, once-a-day oral pimozide or sulpiride may be preferable for maintenance because of fewer side-effects.

Patients with schizophrenia are often incompletely aware of their illness or are indifferent to it. Consequently they may be careless about taking the tablets regularly which are, in fact, beneficial, or they may not ask for a further prescription. They do not come to the doctor, who must seek them out if care is to be maintained; patients tend not to turn up to appointments and, if this happens, doctor, nurse or social worker must go to them at home. Again, this is where a personal relationship is important in achieving continuity of treatment. An attendance each month at a clinic where such relationships can be fostered can become a regular matter.

The care of schizophrenics is a long-term job which should not be regarded as a simple routine for a community nurse or a succession of junior doctors. While these staff play an important part, there must also be regular four- to six-monthly medical reviews by the responsible consultant. Often, it is only the consultant and general practitioner who are able to provide continuity of care over many years of illness. This is because patients and their illnesses evolve and slowly change and the effects on them of drugs alter. Their families and friends should be regularly asked about their performance.

In or out of hospital, the general management of schizophrenics should try to meet their disabilities. Regular encouragement and moderate stimulation keep them from lapsing too far into inertia. They need human relationships but not very demanding ones, whether in work or domestic life. Emotional stress predisposes to further breakdowns and young schizophrenics may do better away from home. The families of schizophrenics often need a good deal of advice and support and this, also, is part of further treatment.

Long-term use of phenothiazines or butyrophenones requires careful consideration. They can produce harmful effects, tardive dyskinesia for instance, and may have doubtful therapeutic effect. On the other hand, a schizophrenic illness can be so devastating that it is justifiable to go to great lengths to prevent or minimise it. A single attack of acute schizophrenia will not usually justify long-term drug treatment, whereas two attacks two years or less apart, or three attacks in five years almost certainly will.

Obviously, the patient whose hallucinations and paranoid outbursts are controlled by drugs should continue to take drugs. A problem arises in the chronically disabled person, predominantly lacking in energy or feeling, whose residual symptoms are not helped appreciably by drugs. Should they be on long-term treatment? The answer lies in deciding whether their state is static, in which case long-term drugs are of no value, or whether their history shows episodes of worsening – patches of bizarre or disturbed behaviour or increased vagueness or bewilderment, for instance – in which case long-term treatment may be helpful. Maintaining medication long term appears to allow many schizophrenics to function better and to prevent relapses. Depot clinics and regular supervision by community psychiatric nurses are key parts of treatment but regular assessment, as to the level of drug and possible side-effects, are essential. If patients are stable, drugs may be reduced gradually, at about three-monthly intervals (see p. 174). On or off medication, it is probably desirable for schizophrenics to be seen regularly.

Current practice leads to many schizophrenic patients, with continuing impairment, living in the community. They are vulnerable to exploitation and social pressures, may have difficulty in making friends or finding social entertainment, are often poor at looking after their own domestic and business interests, failing to shop and cook for themselves, or to claim money to which they are entitled. Collaboration with voluntary bodies such as the National Schizophrenia Fellowship can provide a network of support and advice to patients and their relatives. A clinic should keep a register of all schizophrenic patients in its area, whether resident or coming and going, marking the dates they are seen and issuing reminders for fresh contact. At the same time a balance has to be struck between interference in the life of the disabled and encouragement to further independence. Patients discharged from hospital often take time to recover their full capacity for self-government. On the other hand, there have been too many examples of schizophrenics sinking without trace.

11 Extrapyramidal reactions

Extrapyramidal reactions are an important side-effect of psychotropic drugs, especially phenothiazines and butyrophenones and, more rarely, high-dose tricyclics and lithium. These neurological side-effects should be recognised by psychiatrists but may not be by clinicians in other specialties. Signs vary from the barely noticeable to the very obvious. Four types of reaction are described: acute dystonia, akathisia, Parkinsonism, which occur early in the course of treatment, and tardive dyskinesia, which develops later.

Acute dystonia is a painless, although often frightening, spasmodic involuntary contraction of one or more muscle groups, and comes on suddenly. The patient may writhe, twist and protrude the tongue. Spasm of the muscles of the jaw, neck, spine and eyeball can occur and cause trismus, torticollis, opisthotonos or an oculogyric crisis, depending on the muscle groups affected. So bizarre are these symptoms that hysteria can be mistakenly diagnosed. The patient may present as an emergency in casualty, or it may be an alarming new symptom in the course of a psychiatric illness. The reaction occurs early in the course of drug treatment, sometimes after the first dose.

Akathisia is the name given to a compulsive motor restlessness, especially of the legs, usually accompanied by an unpleasant sense of mental agitation. This discourages patients from taking neuroleptics. The name means an inability to sit down, reflected in the term 'the jitters'. A patient with akathisia will stand, leaning against a wall, alternately lifting one leg and then the other or, when sitting down, cross and uncross the legs with greater than usual frequency. The continual activity and apprehension can mislead, so that more drug, not less, is prescribed for control. Akathisia is a common sight in the settings where the long-term mentally ill are treated.

Parkinsonism resembles post-encephalitic Parkinson's disease in excessive salivation and seborrhoea. Because the cause is a drug effect, the term 'pseudo-Parkinsonism' is sometimes used. Tremor, unusual early on, becomes commoner later. Severity varies from the barely perceptible absence of facial expression and stiffness of posture or gait to complete immobility. Drug-induced Parkinsonism is the most frequently encountered of the extrapyramidal reactions. Weeks may elapse between the start of drug treatment and symptom onset. The diagnosis is readily overlooked, the clinical picture being mistaken for schizophrenic apathy or depression. Some degree of Parkinsonism may have to be tolerated because of the drug doses required to maintain control of a psychosis.

Tardive dyskinesia occurs sometimes only after years of neuroleptic treatment. Involuntary movements of choreiform or athetoid type affect the orofacial muscles, and sometimes the trunk and limbs, resulting in abnormal posture and gait, sometimes grotesque in severity. Smacking of the lips, grimacing, tongue protrusion, grunting and blepharospasm are often striking. Old age, brain damage and female sex appear to predispose to tardive dyskinesia. Some cases appear to result from the brain disorders underlying psychoses rather than from neuroleptic drugs. The range of disordered movement suggests more than one condition; the single term, 'tardive dyskinesia', does not indicate a true entity.

Differential diagnosis

Anxiety, agitation and depression can be excluded with greater certainty if the doctor is aware that the patient either has taken recently, or continues to receive, a drug that can produce extrapyramidal signs as a side-effect. Hysteria, encephalitis, Parkinson's disease, Sydenham's chorea and Huntington's chorea may be diagnosed in error. Trismus, or 'lock jaw', may suggest tetanus, and tardive dyskinesia may resemble a slow form of tetanus. The almost complete relaxation of the affected muscles between spasms and during sleep, the entire absence of pain, and the normal movement of muscles, other than those subject to spasms, are the main features that distinguish the drug-induced condition from tetanus.

A real danger is the prescription of more phenothiazine to control side-effects, mistaking them for partly controlled mental illness. If in doubt about whether the signs are those of mental illness or drug side-effect, reduce or even stop the drug and observe.

Treatment

Dystonic reactions can be reversed in 15 minutes or so by 1–2 mg of benztropine, or 10 mg procyclidine given intravenously or intramuscularly, followed by oral procyclidine, benztropine, benzhexol or orphenadrine until full control is established. Akathisia can usually be controlled or lessened with these oral anticholinergic drugs. Should they fail, benzodiazepines may relieve the distressing mental agitation.

An attempt to control or lessen Parkinsonism by altering dose frequency or dose reduction of neuroleptic should be tried before prescribing anti-Parkinsonian drugs. For example 25 mg fluphenazine decanoate every two weeks could be given weekly as 12.5 mg, which reduces peak levels in the body; or the period between doses extended to three or four weeks. Dose reduction of neuroleptic carries a risk of relapse of mental illness. Only if distressing Parkinsonian symptoms persist after dose adjustment need anticholinergic drugs be prescribed. L-dopa and amantadine, valuable in Parkinson's disease, do not relieve drug-induced Parkinsonism.

Long-term phenothiazine treatment, especially in high dosage, can cause tardive dyskinesia. If early signs appear, stop the phenothiazine and see if the signs go. Sometimes they worsen before diminishing. But dose reduction increases the risk of relapse, which must be balanced against the disability of the dyskinesia. Tetrabenazine (75–200 mg a day) may help with control but can cause depression. Frequent review of the need for long-term and high-dosage phenothiazines is therefore good practice. Thioridazine and sulpiride are said to carry less risk of tardive dyskinesia than other neuroleptics.

With depot injections, anticholinergic drugs may be needed for only a few days immediately after each depot injection when neuroleptic serum levels are briefly increased. Here the patient may be the best judge of need, dose and dose frequency. Intramuscular anticholinergic drug with the depot injection, an alternative to oral drug, gives cover for 24 to 48 hours after the depot injection.

Routine prescribing of anticholinergic drugs at the commencement of treatment with neuroleptics is undesirable because not all patients treated with neuroleptics develop extrapyramidal reactions. The possibility of harm from long-term anticholinergic medication has not yet been excluded and drug dependency, encouraged by the 'buzz' experienced by a few patients (with desire for higher doses), occurs in some. Tolerance to neuroleptics does develop and then anticholinergic drugs may no longer be required. Their gradual withdrawal, by several dose reductions, should be tried from time to time; sudden withdrawal may provoke more severe Parkinsonian symptoms as the nervous system has developed some physical dependence.

12 Acute and chronic brain syndromes

Acute brain syndrome is also called 'dysmnesic syndrome', 'toxic confusional state', 'acute confusion', or 'delirium'. Chronic brain syndrome, commonest in the elderly, is also termed 'brain damage' or 'dementia'. Since the chronic syndrome predisposes to attacks of the acute syndrome both occur most often in old people, although they can occur at any age.

Impairment of memory and other intellectual functions, degrees of disorientation in time and place or even person, partial loss of awareness, perceptual disorders and a general lessening in self-care, with an increased self-centredness, are key signs of brain dysfunction from organic disease. The signs may be mild, moderate, or severe, and may fluctuate from day to day. They may come on gradually and persist, or acutely and be largely or completely reversible. Sometimes an acute attack is superimposed on a chronic illness as yet so mild as to be hardly noticeable.

The two syndromes arise from many physical causes, and every case requires a careful physical examination and appropriate laboratory tests to try to discover the cause. Treatment has three aims: control of symptoms if these are troublesome; management of the underlying causal condition, if identified; and the long-term management of residual symptoms and handicaps.

Acute brain syndrome

Patients with confusional symptoms of recent acute onset often present during treatment for some other condition – medical, surgical or psychiatric – in the home, in casualty or in hospital. Patients in intensive care or after eye operations are particularly liable to become confused.

If patients are restless, noisy, frightened, aggressive or unable to co-operate in their care, immediate physical treatment may be essential before the definite cause has been identified. Chlorpromazine (100–200 mg intramuscularly, repeated every four hours), or haloperidol (5–10 mg intramuscularly or intravenously, repeated in two hours), may be required to achieve rapid control, that is within three or four hours (see p. 177). In milder cases, diazepam (20 mg intramuscularly or intravenously four-hourly) may be sufficient.

Nursing care of confused patients is important. Nurses must identify themselves positively and make themselves known, by touch as well as voice, each time they do something for the patient.

After 24 hours it should be possible to reduce the drug dosage and then to stop altogether in two or three days without return of symptoms. Most deliria and other acute syndromes are short-lasting and resolve spontaneously in three to ten days even without drug treatment but regular daily assessments are needed. (When drugs are ineffective or cannot be used, electroconvulsive therapy (ECT) is an alternative which will bring an acute brain syndrome under control: one treatment is usually enough.)

Patients whose acute syndrome takes a quieter path – an episode of partial disorientation and muddle, unexpected bedwetting, some strange behaviour, a sudden hallucinosis – may best be left without any drug treatment, simply nursed and observed.

When searching for a cause, prescribed drugs should be suspected and stopped if medically possible. In the general medical ward digoxin or pentazocine, for example, may be responsible for an acute brain syndrome. In the psychiatric ward imipramine, amitriptyline, chlorpromazine, benzhexol, lithium, benzodiazepines and tranylcypromine are examples of commonly used psychotropic drugs that can provoke an acute brain syndrome, sometimes when the dose is excessive and sometimes in the recommended dose recently started.

Individuals vary greatly in their susceptibility to produce toxic blood levels while taking the usual dose. Poor renal performance, for instance, reduces clearance of the drug and impaired liver function interferes with the removal of the drug and its derivatives by metabolism. And sometimes the delirium may be an inexplicable response to therapeutic blood levels.

In the young, experimentation with euphoriants, illicit drugs or hallucinogenic plants may produce delirium and is the commonest cause in this age group. Urine screening will identify some of these drugs. Dependence on barbiturates or alcohol may cause delirium if the customary drug intake is not kept up, for example following admission to hospital. Patients may not reveal what they feel to be a shameful habit, making the diagnosis that much harder.

Serious infection with a fever, even mild infections in the elderly, congestive heart failure, anaemia and renal failure may be physical causes of a brain syndrome. An excess of ECT can lead to persisting confusion for a limited period.

To discover the causal disease may require a search for subdural haematoma, a cerebrovascular accident, an endocrine disturbance, or recognition of an unadmitted drug overdose (suicidal?). When the symptoms of the acute syndrome have cleared and the underlying cause of the attack found, if it is possible to do that, and treated, make sure there is no residual mental deficit. The acute attack may have been made more likely because of a gradually developing chronic brain syndrome which needs attention.

A new cause of delirium is the acquired immune deficiency syndrome (AIDS), because of cerebral effects. The principles outlined are still appropriate for the control of an acute brain syndrome in a patient with AIDS. A complication arises from the danger to staff of infection from an uncooperative patient.

Chronic brain syndrome

The progressive loss of faculties, often behind a facade of politeness and social facility which hides deterioration, must be distinguished from the pseudodementing depression of the elderly. Pseudodementia responds to antidepressant drugs or ECT or, temporarily, to a night of complete sleep deprivation; chronic brain syndrome is not reversible unless its physical cause is treatable and found early. The cause of chronic brain syndrome is usually the senile form of cerebral degeneration of the Alzheimer type. Less often the damage is the result of cerebrovascular disease. Other, less common causes include chronic inflammatory conditions, the effects of trauma, degenerative disorders like Creutzfeldt–Jakob disease and Huntington's disease. These conditions are not treatable. Subdural haematomas, benign cerebral tumours such as meningiomas and possibly 'normal-pressure hydrocephalus' can be treated successfully.

In practice, an energetic diagnostic search is made only in those patients in whom, by youth or history of rapid onset or distinctive clinical picture, a senile or multi-infarct dementia seems unlikely. To investigate fully every elderly person with a dementing syndrome is not practical.

Depressive feelings and illnesses

Patients with brain damage sometimes show fluctuating mood swings, anxiety, irritability, or feelings of depression secondary to themselves recognising, if only in part, their disabled state. This lability of mood must not be mistaken for a depressive illness for it does not respond to antidepressant medication or to ECT and may be made much worse if they are used. In a rare variant, the patient may have attacks of weeping without actually feeling miserable at all; these attacks may be lessencd with small doses of thioridazine or chlorpromazine. Occasionally patients with focal brain damage, or strokes, may develop a depressive illness responsive to antidepressants.

Management

The patient with a damaged brain is more sensitive to psychotropic drugs and so requires them in smaller quantities to avoid toxic effects. When such a patient is admitted, a wise move is to stop all psychotropic drugs, review the usefulness of the others, and observe whether the mental state improves.

Insomnia should be tackled by general methods before resorting to hypnotics. A regular routine, hot milk at night, avoidance of indigestion, constipation or nocturia by means of a sensible diet, attention to the warmth and weight of the bed-clothes and height of the pillows, and so on, may solve the problem (see also pp. 33–35).

Improving the patient's bodily health may have an impressive effect on mental state and behaviour. Urinary infection, gastrointestinal upset and respiratory infections may need to be treated. More serious medical conditions such as diabetes or cardiac failure may be uncovered by an appropriate medical assessment.

However, in spite of such measures, restlessness, especially at night, irritability and insomnia may require drug treatment. Thioridazine (25–50 mg) or promazine (25 mg twice daily and/or at night) may be effective. The generally benign benzodiazepines are less safe. They are potent causes of ataxia and delirium in the elderly, while barbiturates and bromides (sometimes in over-the-counter medicines) have a terrible, justified reputation for causing confusional states and are contraindicated. Any psychotropic drug in bigger doses may cause incontinence and falls, even before confusion.

There is no scientific evidence that so-called 'cerebrovascular vasodilators' improve cerebral function significantly. Acetylcholine precursors or cholinesterase inhibitors have so far not proved worthwhile either. Vitamins should only be prescribed where the patient has had an inadequate diet for some time, has had a gastrectomy or other interference with intestinal function, or has frank symptoms of a vitamin deficiency with laboratory evidence justifying the diagnosis. The long-term management of patients with chronic brain syndrome includes the encouragement of physical independence, and the exercise of the remaining intellectual and social faculties, through provision of suitable occupations. Simple tasks can improve the quality of life of patients with dementia, and simple group techniques and clear labelling of rooms, etc., can increase reality orientation.

13 Disorders of childhood

Many psychological disturbances are a normal part of development. Transient fears of strangers, animals and imaginary monsters are all appropriate at certain ages; a degree of defiance and recklessness is an expected part of the acquisition of independence. Parents or teachers rather than the child present the complaint; referrals to a clinic may therefore stem from the difficulties of a depressed, obsessional, inexperienced or rejecting adult in coping with an essentially normal child. Assessment must therefore be directed to the child's home and school as well as to the individual child. The child psychiatrist is the person to do this and plan treatment.

Whether a child needs treatment is based on an evaluation of the following features:

(a) the duration of symptoms: a short-lived tendency to isolation during a time of stress might wisely be regarded as benign and self-limiting; persistent and prolonged social withdrawal probably means something is wrong
(b) the developmental stage of the child: wetting the bed in a four-year-old is probably not an indication for treatment but in a ten-year-old it very likely is
(c) the number and severity of symptoms: minor rituals and compulsions are unremarkable, but pervasive and severe obsessions causing suffering need treatment
(d) the handicap which the symptoms impose on normal psychological development.

Usually the important consideration is (d), and it requires an understanding of the major influences for good and ill in a child's life. Hyperkinetic behaviour in a child from a normal home may disrupt relationships and warrant treatment with stimulant drugs, while for a child in a deprived environment overactivity may be the only way to get adult attention.

The place of drugs

A decision to use drugs as a part of the treatment plan is usually taken by the child psychiatrist and depends on whether the symptoms are likely to be suppressed by a drug, the side-effects of the drug and the chances of getting the same or better results with psychological treatments alone. Also, drugs treat symptoms and will not alter fundamental pathological processes.

In general, be slower to prescribe for children than for adults. Nevertheless, serious psychiatric symptoms are such a barrier to normal development that, when psychological or social treatments are ineffective, useful medication must not be withheld for ideological reasons.

Drugs should only be given for definite indications and are uncommon in clinical practice. Drugs should be given as one part of a management programme, supported by careful explanation and by discouragement of any tendency for the child or the parents to place the responsibility for the child's conduct on the drug. Many parents, teachers and social workers react with such suspicion to the introduction of a drug that a sensitive and understanding discussion of its value is required to encourage co-operation and ensure that the child gets what is prescribed.

The effects of psychotropic drugs are not as well known for children as they are for adults. Children metabolise most drugs more rapidly than adults and the dose response differs from that of adults. Also, what the drug is to do in the child may differ from what it does in adults. For these reasons, it is not safe to calculate the child's dose from the adult dose corrected for body weight. Start the drug in a low dose and then assess the effects of increasing the dose gradually.

The commonest indications for psychotropic drug prescription are nocturnal enuresis, disorders of sleep, hyperactivity, depression and anxiety, conduct problems in the retarded, and symptoms of childhood psychosis.

Nocturnal enuresis

Most children who wet the bed do not come for treatment. Indeed, bedwetting does not usually get medical intervention before the age of six years, at which age 80% of children are dry. Some children are ashamed of wetting and distressed by their apparent weakness; for others bedwetting is a focus for rejection by exasperated parents.

Nocturnal enuresis itself is usually simple to treat; there need be no hesitation on the grounds that treating a symptom will worsen an underlying psychiatric condition. Rather, abolition of enuresis is likely to improve the child's sense of well-being. Initial assessment should include identifying other problems, appraising the child's psychological strengths and weaknesses and those of the family. If micturition is normal in the daytime and no abnormality is found on physical examination, neurological investigations need not be done. Urine should be cultured, especially in girls, and any infection investigated and treated.

A record of dry and wet nights is then kept by child and parent in the form of a star chart. Sometimes this is sufficient treatment. The most effective treatment and the safest is the enuresis alarm: the child soon learns to wake and pass urine when the bladder is full. If the alarm fails or is impractical due to family circumstances, such as overcrowding, then tricyclic antidepressants in low doses can be tried. Their action is rapid; they usually reduce wetting within a week. Relapse, however, is common when treatment is stopped.

Tricyclics can be toxic: they should not be given lightly nor to exceptionally young children. A special hazard is accidental overdose of the palatable elixir by very young children. If there are other young children in the house precautions must be taken against them taking the medicine themselves.

The three-year-old is particularly vulnerable. If drug treatment is to be prolonged then cardiovascular status should be monitored.

If the disability from the enuresis justifies prescription, then imipramine in a dose of 0.5–1.5 mg/kg is suitable; if 50 mg given two hours before bed is not effective, there is no point in trying higher doses. Imipramine probably works by an unidentified central effect separate from its antidepressant and peripheral effects. If a tricyclic fails to work, more complex behavioural approaches for teaching continence are available.

Sleep disorders

Simple sleeplessness is often transient, requiring little intervention. The disturbance to parents may be much greater than any to the child. It is usually a better goal that the wakeful child should play quietly in its own room than that the usual hours of sleep should be extended by hypnotics. However, when an established sleep rhythm has been disrupted, for example by a period of distress, a short course of hypnotic drug may be useful.

Short-acting drugs are preferable. Unfortunately, all are likely to exert a sedative action the next morning and so impair learning ability. Chloral in a dose of 40 mg/kg is usually effective, and its half-life of eight hours is shorter than that of the benzodiazepines so often prescribed.

Night-terrors are to be distinguished from nightmares. In night-terrors, the child wakes confused and in a panic from deep sleep and does not remember the episode. Night-terrors have no sinister significance but may be associated with other rather benign problems of stage IV sleep such as sleep-walking. Reassurance for the parents is usually all that is required. When night-terrors do cause suffering or handicap diazepam in a dose of 0.1–0.3 mg/kg will reduce the frequency by diminishing the proportion of time spent in stage IV sleep.

Hyperactivity

Many children are boisterous and energetic and may be described as overactive by harried caretakers, but these are not grounds for formal diagnosis or treatment. The few children who are chaotic and ill-regulated in their behaviour, inattentive to the point where their ability to learn is impaired, need a full psychiatric assessment and possibly treatment. The treatment plan is guided by the pattern of behaviour shown, in part by the psychological and physical causes, insofar as these can be known.

If the chief difficulty is defiant, aggressive and unruly conduct, then behaviour-modification techniques are likely to be at least as effective as drugs, and are usually best presented in combination with family counselling. If the chief difficulty is in poor academic learning, then remedial education is likely to be the most important intervention, with individual counselling also having a part to play in counteracting the sense of failure which may have arisen.

Medication is most helpful when the chief difficulties are inattentive, disinhibited, disruptive behaviour and poor concentration preventing psychological treatments from working. This is regardless of whether brain damage is the cause. The first choice in drug treatment is a stimulant, preferably dexamphetamine in a dose of 0.1–0.5 mg/kg or pemoline (0.5–2.0 mg/kg). The drugs lead to an improvement in the behaviour problems, and to better performance on laboratory tests of sustained attention, motor control and reaction time. These are not paradoxical effects, but similar to those seen in normal adults and intelligent children. A starting dose of 2.5 mg dexamphetamine daily can be doubled after three days and thereafter increased in increments of 2.5 mg to the optimal dose for the individual (see pp. 159–161). Twice- or even thrice-daily dosage may be necessary because of the drug's short half-life. The commonest unwanted effects are appetite suppression and sleep loss, usually transient and dose-related. Growth retardation can take place with long-term, high-dose medication, possibly due to endocrine changes unrelated to appetite suppression. Misery and irritability, especially in those with brain injuries, may be another stimulant side-effect. Stimulants, excepting pemoline, are legally controlled substances. Although addiction has not been reported as a consequence of taking prescribed drugs in therapeutic doses, children may find that they are able to sell their tablets illicitly.

The need for careful monitoring of action is all the greater because different psychological processes respond to different doses of drug: concentration often improves at a lower dose than overactive behaviour. Indeed, a dose which is optimal for restless behaviour may actually lead to deterioration in the ability to attend. Both need to be assessed; the desired goal must be clear. The uncertainties surrounding the use of stimulants are emphasised by the enormous difference in practice between the USA, where more than half a million children receive such drugs, and the UK where this treatment is given exceptionally. Benzodiazepines should be avoided: they are useless and sometimes harmful. Major tranquillisers can control wildly overactive behaviour when stimulants fail, but this is usually at the price of damaging the ability to learn. Low-dose haloperidol (0.02–0.08 mg/kg) is preferred. Tricyclic antidepressants in low dosage of 1.0 mg/kg have an effect very similar to that of the stimulants but with a higher incidence of side-effects, especially cardiovascular ones.

Affective states

Depressive conditions can occur in children before puberty, but presentation can differ from that in adults. In children, aggressive and defiant conduct, decline in school performance, and underlying pains may indicate depression. The place of antidepressant medication is therefore controversial.

A conservative approach is to prescribe antidepressants, say imipramine in a dose of 50–125 mg daily, only when the symptoms of depression as seen in adults are present and psychological treatment has failed or is impractical.

Similar medication can be advised for refractory school refusal, in combination with family counselling and graded reintroduction to classroom study.

Monoamine oxidase inhibitors have little value for children, especially since dietary precautions can be impossible to maintain. Benzodiazepines are seldom effective in reducing anxiety, and carry the hazard of impairing concentration and learning.

Psychosis

The symptoms of infantile autism place a serious handicap upon a child, and are usually rather static. A painstaking and lengthy educational approach has most to offer, and most parents will need support in coping with the difficulties of care. Neuroleptic treatment has a small but definite role in controlling agitation and stereotyped repetitive behaviour, which it can do in relatively low dose (e.g. thioridazine 50–100 mg daily).

Bleulerian schizophrenia, occasionally seen in pre-pubertal children, can be overdiagnosed if one fails to appreciate the frequency in normal childhood of some blurring between fantasy and reality. When hallucinations or delusions are present, then their control with phenothiazines or other neuroleptics follows similar principles to those governing adult treatment. Children seem to be more prone than adults to dyskinesia but less likely to develop Parkinsonian symptoms.

Conduct disorders in the retarded

The approach to prescribing for the mentally retarded is discussed in the following chapter. Large doses of neuroleptics sometimes quieten aggression but carry high risks of causing movement disorders, especially in the brain damaged. Large doses also reduce attention and learning, crucial abilities in all children and especially so in the impaired child. Surveys show that, in spite of these hazards, long-term, high-dose phenothiazines are prescribed for a large proportion of mentally retarded, psychotic children in institutions. This practice is not sound. Behavioural programmes usually achieve good results without medication. However, some handicapped children express their psychoses and mood disorders with altered behaviour: aggression is the most troublesome. Here careful use of phenothiazines, antidepressants, carbamazepine or lithium can further behavioural and social programmes of care.

Paediatric doses

Titration of dose against response is the soundest way of prescribing. The doses recommended here are guides to decide a starting dose based on milligrams per kilogram of body weight. Individual differences in children at each age are so great that weight is a better guide to dose than age. The approximate average weight of a 6-year-old child is 20 kg (3 st 3 lb), a 10-year-old 30 kg (4 st 10 lb) and a 15-year-old 50 kg (7 st 12 lb).

The following dose/weight schedule is a guide.

Imipramine, 0.5–1.5 mg/kg for enuresis; 1.5–3.5 mg/kg for depression.

Dexamphetamine, 0.1–0.5 mg/kg, pemoline, 0.5–2.0 mg/kg for hyperactivity.

Thioridazine, 1.5–3.5 mg/kg, chlorpromazine, 1.5–3.5 mg/kg for psychoses.

Haloperidol, 0.02–0.08 mg/kg for hyperactivity; 0.1–0.5 mg/kg for control of psychotic symptoms.

14 Mental retardation

Impairment of mental development from birth or the early years may be called 'mental deficiency', 'mental handicap' or 'mental retardation'. 'Mental handicap' is now commonly used in Britain to label those needing special services, but 'mental retardation' is the preferred term, used internationally. One individual may have it in mild degree, another moderately, another severely. In some (but not all) it is associated with structural abnormality of the brain, and this 'damage' or deficiency may be generalised or localised. It is commonest among the severely retarded, one-third of whom also suffer from epilepsy. Over half of these people will need anticonvulsants at some time in their lives.

Mentally handicapped people are more likely than other people to suffer from mental illnesses. Of those admitted to mental handicap hospitals 6% suffer from manic–depressive or schizophrenic illnesses, and some of the other behaviour disorders – hyperkinetic syndrome and autism in children, hysterical reactions and anxiety states in adults – may benefit from drug treatment as part of their management. The mentally retarded person is more easily upset than the normal person by difficulty and frustration: lessening anxiety and irritability may reduce ritualistic behaviour or temper outbursts.

Always try to understand the patient's behaviour, and never simply to suppress it. As also emphasised elsewhere in this book, always prescribe drugs for specific indications or with specific purposes in mind, usually for a clearly limited period only, and never on grounds of general indefinite sedation. An acutely disturbed person may be sedated temporarily as a way of breaking up a fraught situation and starting again from a calm baseline with a programme of social contacts, reassurance, and occupation. An anxious person may be helped by a regular anxiolytic, a person with a depressive illness by a tricyclic antidepressant (see Chapters 8, 9, 21, 26). Repeated explosive outbursts may respond to lithium carbonate or carbamazepine. The epileptic will require anticonvulsants. But there are many mentally handicapped individuals who do not require drugs at all. Where they do, remember to adjust doses to the age and size of the person, whether child or old man, just as for the non-handicapped. Drug treatment should not be used by itself, but as part of a thought-out programme of behavioural management, psychotherapy of some type, and environmental manipulation.

Two special points must be mentioned. One is that structural brain abnormality, or damage, can alter drug responses. It is therefore best to be cautious with size of doses, until experience with a person has taught what is possible. Barbiturates in particular may make irritable rather than sedate, so that phenobarbitone or primidone may be unsuitable as anticonvulsants: phenytoin or carbamazepine will be preferable. The other is to remember that mentally retarded persons may not be good at learning to manage their own tablet-taking, or at reporting its effects to the doctor. It is therefore very important to involve parents and relatives, social workers and nurses, in the drug treatment plan from the beginning, so that they can agree with or question what is being attempted and help to further its successful outcome. Of course, the patients, particularly in the community, should also be involved: they may need a special training programme on how to manage their own drugs.

15 Epilepsy

Most people with epilepsy live stable lives without serious mental symptoms. Of those epileptics seen by psychiatrists, about one in six of the total, some will be resident in long-stay hospitals for the mentally ill or mentally retarded or in 'epileptic colonies', but many will be living independently. Of those seen, a small proportion are diagnostic problems, others are chronic sufferers from epilepsy who also have to contend with something added: neurotic symptoms, personality difficulties, a psychosis, or the effects of brain damage and impaired intellect. It is these added conditions that have brought them to psychiatric attention.

The purpose of this section is to assist the psychiatrist to assess and manage the drug treatment of fits.

Diagnosis

Inexplicable episodes of aggression, irritability or other behaviour disturbance, bizarre sensations, panics, amnesias, disorientations, or 'absences' are not necessarily epileptic and may result from psychiatric disorders such as early schizophrenia, neurosis, hysteria or a personality disorder. But they may be evidence of petit mal or temporal lobe epilepsy. Careful description of the behaviour and the abnormal mental experience, possibly a period of observation in hospital, and an electroencephalogram (EEG) may be required to decide.

Major fits may occur in catatonic schizophrenia, in dementia, as an early or late effect of brain injury, after a leucotomy, in alcoholism and other drug addictions, and as a result of excessive drinking of water. A fit can result from a tricyclic antidepressant, phenothiazine, barbiturate, benzodiazepine or other psychotropic drug. Tricyclics and many neuroleptics lower fit threshold, predisposing non-epileptic patients to seizures. Rapid dose reduction of sedative drugs (as by sudden omission of scheduled doses of benzodiazepines or barbiturates for example) may provoke a fit, especially if the drugs have been taken for a long time. An isolated fit may therefore be a drug effect.

Epileptics well controlled on drugs may have unexpected fits or a change in fit pattern. Occasional failure to take anticonvulsant drugs, or taking drugs which change anticonvulsant drug metabolism, or an increase in alcohol intake, or psychological distress and sleep deprivation may all alter fit threshold. A few epileptics learn how to induce fits and some have 'hysterical' fits. Distinguishing between true and hysterical or simulated fits may be assisted by the serum prolactin which is temporarily increased after a true fit but not after a hysterical one. But many drugs, especially neuroleptics, raise the prolactin level and obscure this test.

Drug treatment

A single fit is not necessarily epilepsy. Never give an anticonvulsant drug after only one fit. Look, first, for a medical or neurological cause or a drug effect, and treat this if it is possible to do so. Only prescribe anticonvulsants when these causes have been excluded, where fits are recurring and the patient is embarrassed or in danger thereby.

The aim is to stop all fits using only one drug, and without producing disabling side-effects. In practice this ideal cannot be achieved with everyone, but seizures can be controlled completely in over one-half of treated epileptics with only mild side-effects; and another third have fit frequency or severity diminished (see p. 206).

The choice of drug depends on the type of seizure. For generalised tonic–clonic fits carbamazepine or phenytoin are the drugs of choice. Carbamazepine is preferred because phenytoin is sedative, can cause hirsutism, coarsening of the face, and gum hypertrophy. Where carbamazepine and phenytoin fail, sodium valproate, primidone or phenobarbitone can be tried. The last two are sedative and cause irritability and restlessness. Prefer phenobarbitone always.

Partial fits should be treated in the same way as generalised seizures. Temporal lobe fits are treated with carbamazepine. Petit mal attacks respond to ethosuximide or sodium valproate or, if these fail, clonazepam. Clonazepam is sedative and can aggravate disorderly behaviour. Atypical 'absence seizures' in secondary generalised epilepsy and myoclonic epilepsies are difficult to control but the same drugs should be tried.

Commence treatment in the new case with a low dose of the chosen drug. If after a week evidence of response is lacking increase the dose by small increments every few days until fits cease, early side-effects, especially drowsiness, become intolerable or measurement of the serum level shows the concentration of drug to be at the top of the therapeutic range. For infrequent fits this assessment obviously takes longer.

If fits still occur with one drug in high dose, add a second, still with the aim of using a single drug in the long-term. Start the second drug in a low dose, increasing the dose in small increments while maintaining the dose of the first. When control is achieved, reduce the dose of the first in small steps with the objective of stopping it. If fits reappear the two drugs will have to be used together. More than two drugs should not be used. The enemy of therapy is sedation, which can be reduced or avoided by using lower doses and the less sedative drug.

Epileptics who continue to have fits in spite of medication may not have the intelligence or the personality to co-operate in treatment. Some may not take their drugs at all and others irregularly. Relatives may know and should be consulted. Serum drug levels are a useful check.

Personality and epilepsy

A chronic and stigmatising disorder such as epilepsy predisposes to episodic irritability and moodiness; failures breed resentment, feelings of inadequacy and of being at the whim of fate. Patients can become religiose, or excessively suspicious of others, and inflexible in their thoughts and attitudes. Drugs such as chlorpromazine or thioridazine can be used to diminish the more disruptive, irritable, aggressive and paranoid symptoms but may lower seizure threshold; carbamazepine can be effective here. But psychological support and social help including sheltered workshops are a good approach.

When fits continue and are apparently difficult to control, in spite of apparent optimal medication, review all drugs taken including those prescribed for conditions other than epilepsy. Perhaps the number of drugs or their dose can be reduced with a reduction of side-effects and without increasing fit frequency. Changes must be made slowly, to avoid the risk of temporarily increasing seizure frequency. Sometimes fit frequency may drop after an initial rise, if the reduced dosage is maintained.

Avoid combinations of drugs with similar actions, for instance primidone with phenobarbitone. Preparations of tablets or capsules containing more than one anticonvulsant drug (no longer available in Britain) should not be used because separate dose adjustment of the constituents is impossible.

Future outlook

Like everyone else, people with epilepsy have spells of anxiety or even depressive illnesses which can be treated in the usual way. Temporal lobe epilepsy carries a risk of a paranoid schizophrenic illness. This can be treated with phenothiazines. Neuroleptic and antidepressant drugs may alter plasma levels of anticonvulsants. Epileptics free of fits for three years and without EEG evidence of epileptic activity may try a slow reduction of their anticonvulsant drugs over three months with the aim of stopping them. One in three may be able to do without medication. A trial without drugs should not be tried if a seizure is likely to pose a risk to others, to the patient, or carry a social cost. Avoid sudden withdrawal of drugs because of the risk of precipitating a sharp increase in fit frequency or status epilepticus.

Epilepsy legally precludes driving cars until there has been a fit-free period of two years, or unless fits occur only in sleep. Epilepsy bars the driving of heavy goods or public service vehicles. The sedation from anticonvulsant drugs may make driving vehicles and operating machinery hazardous, especially if the sufferer also takes alcohol.

Anticonvulsant drugs carry an increased risk of teratogenicity. In spite of this, anticonvulsant drugs will need to be continued during pregnancy because of the risk fits pose to both mother and foetus. The metabolic changes during pregnancy and lactation may cause a fall in serum levels of drugs. Blood levels should be monitored often and especially in the later stages of pregnancy. Most drugs can be continued during lactation because their concentration in milk is not enough to affect the infant; phenobarbitone and primidone are exceptions (so is diazepam).

Epilepsy in children

The drug treatment of epilepsy in children follows the same principles as for adults. Children and their parents require counselling about epilepsy, the actual fits and the drugs to control them. Anti-epileptic drugs can interfere with learning and produce irritability and behaviour problems. Plasma levels may show toxic levels which are not clinically apparent in the brain-damaged or intellectually handicapped child (see also pp. 101, 204–213).

Treatment of status epilepticus

Consecutive seizures without recovery of consciousness between fits is called status epilepticus. The generalised convulsive form is life-threatening because of respiratory obstruction, hypoxic brain damage or cardiac arrhythmia.

The management of status epilepticus comprises: (a) securing an airway; (b) protecting the patient from self-injury; (c) controlling seizures with drugs.

Diazepam can be given as an intravenous infusion for continuous treatment. The dose of drug required is decided from response, effect being assessed after each 10 mg of injection. When seizures subside the infusion can be stopped, and restarted on recurrence of fits. Diazepam (200–300 mg) may be given during the course of 24 hours depending on weight, health and fit persistence. Respiratory depression and hypotension can occur with large doses, as can thrombophlebitis at the injection site. Clonazepam and chlormethiazole may also be used in this way. Paraldehyde remains a useful drug given in a dose of 5–10 ml intramuscularly or rectally. Although its effect lasts longer than that of diazepam it is slower to act, and tissue damage may occur if it is injected.

Diazepam can be given by rectal infusion (Stesolid) if an intravenous infusion is impossible. Seizures must be stopped quickly to minimise the risk of brain damage, and if fits do not lessen in, say, half an hour, with diazepam in a generous dose, the aid of an anaesthetist should be sought. More energetic measures can then be employed while pulmonary and cardiac functions are safeguarded. In children, febrile convulsions lasting more than 15 minutes require hospital treatment as an emergency.

16 Alcoholism

People can enjoy alcoholic drinks and may, on occasion, become drunk without being alcoholics. Alcoholism is a form of drug dependence. Physical dependence is recognised when abstinence for any reason results in the appearance of withdrawal symptoms – tremor or shaking, nausea, weakness, irritability, insomnia. Psychological dependence has no simple set of agreed signs, but displays itself as uncontrolled drinking. Different definitions describe alcoholism in terms of the distress expressed or observed, the damage to physical health, the difficulty in cutting down or giving up drinking altogether, or the damaging effects to working, social or family life.

Alcoholic patients come to psychiatric notice for two reasons: withdrawal symptoms and referral for the treatment of alcoholism. Withdrawal symptoms or even delirium tremens may begin at home, after admission for a non-alcoholic reason to a medical, surgical or psychiatric ward, or after remand in custody, situations where supply of drink is denied. Outpatient referral for treatment of alcoholism is usually on the urging of other people because of the social effects of continuing addiction on the alcoholic or on other people. Sufferers are often unable to give an objectively correct account of the extent of their intake and behavioural disturbance.

Drugs play an important part in detoxification, the treatment of delirium tremens, Wernicke's encephalopathy and the schizophreniform psychosis which a few alcoholics develop. Drugs have only a small part in preserving abstinence from further drinking, where management is largely psychotherapeutic and social.

Attempts to decriminalise drunkenness have resulted in detoxification centres being opened by charities. Management is in the hands of staff especially experienced in treating detoxification, with medical care supplied by general practitioners.

Detoxification

Withdrawal symptoms may be slight or lead to epileptic fits or full-blown delirium tremens. Management often requires hospital admission, especially for the severely affected where there is a risk of death. The principal psychiatric symptoms are insomnia, tremor, weakness, nausea, irritability, confusion, tactile, visual and auditory hallucinations, and terror. Withdrawal fits are common. Acute circulatory collapse, hypothermia and infection may occur and require urgent action. The patient may be dehydrated and hypoglycaemic.

The aim of treatment is the control of psychological symptoms, the prevention of fits, and the care of the patient's physical health. Make sure the patient has no secret supply of alcohol or sedative drugs. Experienced physical nursing and close medical supervision are needed. Temperature, pulse and blood pressure must be noted every four hours and fluid balance recorded. Serum electrolytes and blood glucose need to be checked.

Suppression of psychological symptoms (and prevention of withdrawal fits) can be accomplished with chlordiazepoxide, diazepam or chlormethiazole, the dose depending on age, weight and severity of symptoms: 1 g chlormethiazole every six hours, or 20–40 mg chlordiazepoxide or diazepam every six hours are guide doses. Chlorpromazine or thioridazine (200–600 mg daily) can be also used where disturbance is severe, or 5–10 ml paraldehyde given orally in orange juice or rectally as a saline enema. When symptoms start to wane these drugs should be steadily withdrawn over three to seven days, depending on response. Because heavy drinkers have a poor diet, a course of intramuscular vitamins may be given. In particular, the Wernicke–Korsakov syndrome, arising from lack of thiamine, requires urgent treatment (p. 222).

The sedative drugs used to control symptoms must be reduced and then stopped as soon as withdrawal symptoms are over. Diazepam, chlordiazepoxide and chlormethiazole are, like alcohol, drugs of dependency to the susceptible and should not be used for chronic treatment. Some alcoholics may require small doses of benzodiazepines to help them through the alcohol-free months: this may be preferable to renewed intoxication. With the exception of disulfiram no drugs seem to help in the prevention of relapse, although some patients with chronic depressive features do well with lithium or a tricyclic if they take them regularly.

Assess physical health, looking for malnutrition, infections, peripheral neuritis, and check liver function and test for any signs of an early dementia. Formal psychological memory testing will provide a baseline for the future. Any psychiatric illness must be treated, for instance depression, mania, neurosis.

Although alcoholism, in itself, does not provide grounds for compulsory hospital admission under the Mental Health Act 1983, such action can be appropriate when delirium tremens or a florid psychosis is present.

Prevention of drinking

Alcoholics have to admit to themselves that alcohol is getting the better of them. They must want to regain self-control. They can be helped by recognition of the situations which particularly provoke drinking and by understanding their own self-condemnation and self-punishment. Some people live in particularly predisposing situations, for example, a job which favours a bar life. Social or sexual timidity may be relieved by alcohol. Lack of leisure interests, loneliness at home or bereavement may lead to drinking. Identification of the pattern, and of provoking factors, may lead to helpful changes in lifestyle. For most sufferers, complete abstinence from alcohol in any form must be the target; for a few, very limited moderate drinking may be achievable. Regular contacts over a lengthy period with a friendly doctor, nurse, psychologist or social worker who will be accepting, encouraging and non-judgemental are likely to aid the patient in achieving rehabilitation. Short admissions to hospital at difficult times can be useful in preventing relapses, but most longer-term treatment is now in the community.

Apart from solving the problem of homelessness, a hostel may give valuable support and produce change. Much social help over finance, employment, marriage, loneliness and isolation, and development of new interests may be needed. Special attention must be given to the family. The doctor must be prepared for long-term supervision, for repeated setbacks in some cases, but must never lose heart. Considerable benefit can be expected in two-thirds of cases. The support of fellow sufferers in therapeutic groups, for example the lay society "Alcoholics Anonymous" (AA) (see local telephone directory) helps some.

Some districts have set up alcohol advisory centres which provide a range of information, support and group therapy for alcoholics and their families. These, with AA, are the basis for long-term management.

One marginally useful method of treatment does involve drugs. The patient, who must be in good health, takes disulfiram regularly every morning, possibly under some supervision, for a long period. The drug stops the metabolism of alcohol at the stage of acetaldehyde. Acetaldehyde is a toxic substance producing unpleasant feelings of violent throbbing in the head, dyspnoea, sickness and, in excess, giddiness, failing vision, cardiac irregularity and collapse. The patient on disulfiram learns in hospital that one glass of his favourite drink will provoke unpleasant symptoms, and is thereby helped to avoid the temptation of a single drink when outside (p. 214). However, this only works if the drug is kept up regularly. It is also claimed that lithium carbonate if taken regularly may help abstinence, even in the absence of depressions.

Alcoholic hallucinosis or alcoholic paranoid psychosis responds like schizophrenia to phenothiazines or butyrophenones. Stop all alcohol and give the phenothiazine in suppressive doses (see p. 167). The psychotic state usually clears in a few days. Cautiously reduce drug dose by degrees, and stop altogether when symptoms do not recur. About 10% of patients do not remit and are permanently schizophrenic.

17 Drug dependence

Addiction to drugs or medicines can be divided broadly into three groups, with treatments and prognoses which differ so much as to warrant a separate description of each.

Dependence on soft drugs

Anxiety, tension, worrying, and helplessness, first bring these patients to medical attention. They want regular doses of minor tranquillisers, analgesics, barbiturates or appetite suppressants to avert symptoms and maintain a sense of well-being but they do not become dependent on hard drugs. By the time they reach psychiatric out-patient departments they have usually been provided with drugs for years. Referral is often caused by general practitioners being no longer agreeable to prescribe such drugs long term or patients, themselves influenced by the media emphasising the dangers, wishing to withdraw.

The psychiatrist may decide to advise continuing the supply of drugs, but steps must be taken to ensure that drug intake does not steadily increase, as it may easily do, especially with barbiturates, by agreeing with the family doctor for only one person to prescribe the drug and to fix what the dose shall be. On the other hand, if it is agreed that the aim is withdrawal, appropriate psychological help, usually by group methods, is needed. Which ever course is decided, the longer-term management is a matter for the family doctor.

Stable opiate dependence

A few people become dependent on opiates because of easy access to them or from these 'hard' drugs being overprescribed for the control of pain. If provided with a regular, stable supply of opiates, they can have a reasonably normal life. Indeed, they may suffer hardship if overzealous attempts are made to terminate dependence. The stabilised drug addicts in Britain before 1960 were comprised of this kind. There are not many of them, their numbers are increasing only a little, and they do not often come to the general psychiatrist's attention. When they do, the problem is usually one of stabilising the dosage, which may temporarily have been increased to a harmful level in an attempt to control some increase in stress symptoms.

Unstable opiate dependence

These are the people who present the serious problem for casualty, medical and psychiatric services. They are young, immature, often with serious difficulties in maintaining relationships and work, and consequently with formidable social problems. Their addiction history is of switching from one drug to another, whichever is available, and increasing the amounts taken, all of which brings conflict with the law. Young addicts may dabble with many drugs, having begun with the less toxic. Later they experiment with opiates, for example heroin, diconal, methadone. They begin by taking the drug orally, by inhalation or by intramuscular injection and later learn to use intravenous injections. Stimulants and barbiturates are sometimes added to enhance the effect, which increases the risk of fatal outcome. This kind of polypharmacy is on the increase.

A drug subculture can provide a reasonably stable and satisfying daily life but, even so, there may be accidental or deliberate overdoses, intoxication, infection (including with HIV), abstinence symptoms, acute toxic states and social problems such as domestic crises, homelessness, unemployment, conflict with the law. Drug-taking is usually one symptom of a disturbed personality, and a healthy scepticism in the face of an apparent sudden desire to cease drug-taking is appropriate. The drug may be the only aid the patient now has to maintain a semblance of feeling normal.

Management of withdrawal

This differs, depending on the drug of addiction.

Opiates

Addicts who present themselves unexpectedly at hospital may be concerned to get more drugs, so their stories are unreliable. On the other hand, they may be suffering from the unwanted effects of serious addiction, especially infections, which must be looked for and treated. The management of overdose and infection are not discussed here but withdrawal and long-term treatment are, since those are the psychiatrist's main responsibilities.

Distress and objective signs of withdrawal require treatment, preferably in hospital. Methadone (Physeptone) is the drug of choice and 10–20 mg should be given orally, repeated an hour later if there is no improvement; 40 mg is usually adequate for the first 24 hours. The dose can then be reduced gradually to 5–10 mg a day until the patient is off all opiates. Heroin should not be given, nor is there any need to give other drugs by injection. Clonidine, an anti-hypertensive agent, is used as an alternative to methadone to cover withdrawal. It is claimed to reduce restlessness and somatic withdrawal symptoms especially. But whichever regime is used depends on the agreed policy of a specialist drug unit.

Long-term plans for management will be required which depend heavily on the patient's attitude, since a sustained motivation to terminate dependence is a key factor. A designated treatment centre with experienced staff is the best place to supervise the patient's management; if they cannot accept the patient, the centre will advise.

If there are no signs of withdrawal do not rush into a commitment. Assess the patient and then consult with an expert before offering long-term help. To decide on a plan of treatment may take a week and the patient, if genuine, will wait. Then a form of treatment contract between doctor and patient should be agreed. The detail of the contract will vary depending on the patient, the clinic's facilities and its approach, which should be consistent to all addicts. An example of a contract is to agree to prescribe liquid methadone, for example 20–30 mg a day, and to post the prescription to a local, named, chemist who will supply the drug daily but will not supply more drugs or replace them if they are 'lost'. Then agree to see the patient every week or fortnight for support and to reduce the dose of the drug. Other help such as day hospital, groups, social work, self-help organisations, depend on local facilities and are important ingredients of treatment.

Drug abuse clinics may limit the time of providing regular treatment, for example to three months only, and link this to definite targets. Patients may return again at a later date. Be realistic, but do not accept the constant dose which the patient demands. Encourage reduction. Remember, a too ready prescribing of drugs will rapidly produce a queue of addicts. Urine tests for methadone are of limited value. If positive, they indicate the patient has had the drug less than six hours before; if negative, the patient may not be a genuine addict if withdrawal symptoms are absent, too. The transmission of AIDS by sharing contaminated needles is now a serious problem. Clinics should consider providing clean needles, without charge, to addicts known to inject.

The supply of drugs of addiction to addicts can be given only by practitioners licensed by the Home Office, and the prescriptions must be written in a standard way (see pp. 43, 121). Some National Health Service districts, as policy, restrict licences for prescribing to medical staff of the drug abuse clinic.

Barbiturates

Patients addicted to barbiturates are either multiple drug users, when the barbiturate source is illicit and the drug used to enhance effects of other illicit drugs, or people with chronic sedation or sleeping problems for whom barbiturates have been medically prescribed for years. The size of the second group has slowly lessened with the voluntary agreement of general practitioners not to prescribe barbiturates.

Admission to hospital is required to supervise withdrawal when more than 500–1000 mg daily is being taken. This is to control the serious withdrawal symptoms and avoid a withdrawal psychosis and grand mal fits.

The aim of treatment is first to replace the addictive barbiturates, which are long-acting and slowly removed, with pentobarbitone and then slowly to decrease that drug in a controlled manner. Pentobarbitone is a short-acting and rapidly excreted barbiturate, given to prevent both fits and the less tolerable abstinence symptoms.

One regime is to start 600–1000 mg pentobarbitone a day in four doses. If the patient shows signs of intoxication, one dose is eliminated, but if withdrawal signs are evident a further dose is added. In this way, the dose of pentobarbitone required to stabilise the patient can be achieved in three days. Then, by reducing by 100 mg a day, pentobarbitone can be slowly withdrawn completely. It is best not to use diazepam or phenothiazines during the withdrawal period, which will take from two to three weeks depending on the scale of the addiction.

Even when withdrawal is complete, irritability and sleeplessness may continue for up to three months. The patient should be told and encouraged to tolerate it or relief may be sought with other drugs.

Alternative sedatives are best avoided because the patient may become dependent on another drug. However, it may be practical to give benzodiazepines in small doses for insomnia and daytime sedation for a short time and try to wean the patient from these as well. Dependence on up to 0.5 g barbiturate daily can usually be terminated by out-patient supervision of gradual withdrawal and substitution by benzodiazepines or phenothiazines.

Other drugs

Amphetamines have been used freely by drug users, and in medical practice as appetite suppressants, or antidepressants or energisers, or for narcolepsy. They are not easily obtained now, because of the voluntary ban on their prescription. No physical abstinence syndrome results from stopping small doses, although some psychological support may be required for a short period. Very rarely, a paranoid psychosis occurs but this is from heavy use, not withdrawal, and it will settle without specific treatment when amphetamines are stopped. The patient should be in hospital for this and phenothiazines can be used to suppress symptoms.

Cocaine in large amounts may produce a psychosis similar to amphetamine psychosis; it resolves on withdrawing the drug.

Lysergic acid diethylamide (LSD) is now prescribed rarely but, unofficially, is often used in a single dose to enlarge perceptual experience, sometimes very unpleasantly. Emergency treatment may be required during this so-called 'bad trip', which may cause acute distress or result in the drug-takers harming themselves or others while under the influence of delusions. Experience suggests that management by friends is sufficient, but sometimes it is necessary to terminate the acute psychosis, in which case chlorpromazine (100–200 mg intramuscularly) or diazepam (10–20 mg intravenously) is effective. Quite often the experience is vividly relived later in the so-called 'flash-back'. Drugs are rarely needed unless the 'flash-back' is severe, or is frequent. Phenothiazines, in small amounts, given for a few weeks or months may help. More rarely, a chronic paranoid psychosis resembling schizophrenia occurs, and should be treated with phenothiazines. This may be a schizophrenic illness which could have occurred anyway.

Abuse of Mandrax (methaqualone 250 mg plus diphenhydramine 25 mg) may result in restlessness, anxiety and excitement. Withdrawal needs care to avoid fits. Mandrax is still available illicitly in Britain; although withdrawn from prescription, it is legal in some countries.

Cannabis (Indian hemp), once claimed not to cause psychiatric problems, appears to be associated with schizophrenia-like psychoses and causes relapses of paranoid psychoses. Violent behaviour often occurs and requires high doses of major tranquillisers to control.

The drug scene

Some drug users are now mixing opiates with cannabis and this leads to a highly toxic state. Perhaps a third of heroin users now combine it in mixture with cocaine. Other chemicals are used occasionally and unofficially for their mental effects, especially by the young who are interested in the experience they induce. Only a few people continue taking such drugs regularly and even fewer become addicted, in contrast to alcohol and tobacco. Those who do may suffer from personality problems and it is this group who present to the psychiatrist.

The non-medical use of drugs depends on availability and prevailing popular knowledge of their effects. Many can be obtained over the counter: cough mixtures containing morphine, antihistamine mixtures with codeine, and nasal sprays of isoprenaline, for instance.

There are other substances with an industrial or household use which are sniffed, for example glue, paint thinners, lacquers, some solvents, some aerosols and petrol fumes. They are not dangerous in small amounts and rapidly give a feeling of intoxication. But in large amounts they are dangerous and brain damage and deaths have resulted. Professional people with access can becomc addicted in a similar way to ether, nitrous oxide, cyclopropane, trichloroethylene and other anaesthetic gases. The acute reaction to the inhalation of these drugs requires little medical and no psychiatric care, but the chronic abuser poses the more difficult problems seen in any of the other drug addiction groups, in whom lack of motivation to stop is the most serious. Adhesives are least toxic but some cleaning fluids and aerosols can cause cardiac arrest.

Tobacco and alcohol are the most serious addiction problems today because of their huge mortality and morbidity. Caffeine, probably the most widespread addiction, may not be completely free of harmful effects.

Legal aspects

The Misuse of Drugs Act 1971 was the first step to provide better control over misuse of drugs of all kinds and laid down rules for supply and possession. 'Controlled drugs' are classified in three grades, depending on harmfulness when abused. Penalties for offences are graded similarly.

Class A: examples are cocaine, diamorphine (heroin), dipipanone, LSD, methadone, morphine, opium, pethidine, phencyclidine, and class B drugs when injected
Class B: examples are oral amphetamines, barbiturates, cannabis, codeine, glutethimide, pentazocine, phenmetrazine
Class C: examples are meprobamate, certain drugs related to amphetamines such as benzphetamine and most benzodiazepines.

Further regulations (1973) require details about addicts to be notified to the Home Office. The relevant drugs are cocaine, dextromoramide (Palfium), diamorphine (heroin), dipipanone (Diconal), hydrocodone (Dimotane DC), hydromorphone, levorphanol (Dromoran), methadone (Physeptone), morphine, opium, oxycodone, pethidine, phenazocine (Narphen), piritramide (Dipidolor). If the treating doctor suspects the patient is an addict, that is, is persistently dependent on the drug, the Chief Medical Officer, Home Office Drugs Branch, Queen Anne's Gate, London SW1H 9AT, must be notified within seven days. If the patient is still being treated a year later, a further notification is required. Details have been limited to personal ones and the addictive drug. Since 31 March 1990, a new system operates with more detailed clinical information. This, with personal details, goes, as before, to the Home Office and a copy, without personal identification, goes to local district and regional databases. This will provide data on clients, the use of facilities and a guide to future planning.

The Home Office keeps an index of notified addicts and this is available, on a confidential basis, to doctors. Hence it is wise, when faced by a new addict, to check with the Home Office that the addict is not already being treated elsewhere. Write to the Chief Medical Officer or, more simply, telephone 071-273 2213. The response will be by a return telephone call to ensure the caller is a genuine doctor.

The above applies to England, Scotland and Wales. In Northern Ireland, notification is to the Chief Medical Officer, Ministry of Health and Social Services, Dundonald House, Belfast BT4 3SF, and telephone inquiries to 0232-650111.

A further regulation is that only doctors who hold a special licence from the Home Secretary can prescribe cocaine, diamorphine or dipipanone to drug addicts. In some health districts, it is policy for doctors attached to drug clinics only to hold such licences. This encourages a uniform and consistent approach to treatment. Non-licensed doctors can still prescribe these drugs for relief of severe pain.

Special conditions apply to writing a prescription for controlled drugs. It is to be written in the prescriber's own handwriting, in ink, and include the name and address of the patient, the form and strength of the preparation, the dose, the total quantity of the drug, in words and figures, and be signed and dated.

More advice on the Act and Regulations can be sought from the Regional Senior Inspectors of the Home Office Drugs Branch:

London and the South-East	071-273 3530
The Midlands, South-West England and Wales	0272-276736
Northern England and Scotland	0532-429941

18 Sexual disorders

Complaints of sexual dysfunction occur as the presenting feature of a psychiatric illness, in the course of psychotropic drug treatment, in the setting of a personality problem, and sometimes as a separate source of worry with a request for explanation and reassurance. Some apparently unexplained sexual problems are referred from medical or surgical colleagues because sexual disorders may be considered the psychiatrist's province.

Sexual dysfunction occurs in nearly all psychiatric illness. Depression lowers sexual drive and performance, leading to indifference, impotence or frigidity. In a previously well adjusted couple a serious misunderstanding can result. Explanation of the biological nature of the change and reassurance that normal sexual response will return on recovery from depression usually enables a couple to accept the situation.

Mania, in contrast, heightens sexual drive and sexual enjoyment, the only mental illness to do so. Increased sexual demand in marriage may become a problem for the spouse of a manic patient, and so may promiscuity or sexual deviations. Explanation and reassurance to the well partner assist adjustment but often long-term help is required.

Schizophrenia is associated with low sexual drive which, with deficits in emotional display, limit sexual activity. In early onset, marriage is infrequent and fertility is low. Sexually embarrassing or deviant behaviour occurs sometimes in chronic schizophrenia and may prevent discharge from hospital because of risk of criminal offence. Rarely does serious crime, including homicide, result from paranoid delusions with a sexual content.

Dementia causes serious problems if disinhibited, embarrassing or unlawful sex acts occur. Exposure or other indecency may be the presenting feature, almost exclusively in males.

Alcohol abuse results in loss of sexual drive and ability, as does other substance abuse, but can lead to disinhibition.

Sexual dysfunction arising in these ways usually needs no treatment other than the treatment of the primary psychiatric illness. Embarrassing or potentially criminal sexual conduct occurring in schizophrenia and mental handicap can be dependent on sexual drive and may then respond to drugs which reduce such drive.

The drugs used to treat psychiatric illness often affect sexual function in an unwanted way. Any drug with sedative effect, especially when used in excess, can reduce sexual interest and drive. Neuroleptics, tricyclics and monoamine oxidase inhibitors can cause impotence, delay ejaculation or inhibit it entirely. When tolerance to the drug develops, or the drug is stopped, sexual function usually returns to normal. Many drugs used in general medicine, and which the older psychiatric patient may be taking, also affect sexual function: thiazides, for instance, can cause impotence. Hence the importance of a full drug history.

Sexual dysfunction presenting in the absence of any causal illness requires treatment of sexual performance itself. Sexual problems comprise an increasing part of psychiatric practice because people expect sexual intercourse to be enjoyable and are prepared to do something if it is not. The treatment of primary dysfunction uses a behavioural approach directed at improving the sexual response of a couple to each other. Success depends on motivated, co-operative, sexual partners and a therapist with special skills. Drugs have usually no part in this treatment. Sedative drugs, however, may have a small part to play when anxiety and impotence are linked, especially in the uncertain young man or the overconsciously ageing one. If taken shortly before intercourse, sedative drugs can sometimes improve performance. Drugs are not useful for treating premature ejaculation. In women, dyspareunia, vaginismus and anorgasmia are common complaints leading to worry, resentment, and a poor marital relationship. Drugs are ineffective and may do harm. A behavioural approach is recommended for all these conditions.

A high level of sexual activity, especially if associated with psychopathic personality or sexual deviance, can be a serious problem in men and may result in crime and loss of liberty. Drugs which reduce sexual drive may reduce undesirable conduct. Cyproterone acetate, an anti-androgen which appears to reduce sexual drive, can be effective. The butyrophenone benperidol has been recommended for the reduction of sexual drive but is not of proven value.

When the unwanted behaviour is not sex-drive dependent, as in the older male, drugs which reduce sex drive are not likely to work. Drugs should be combined with psychological treatment aimed at increasing the patient's motivation to alter behaviour and improve self-control. Aside from reduction of anxiety and sexual drive, drugs have little part to play in treating other disorders of sexual function such as homosexuality, fetishism, pederasty, exposure or transvestism.

19 Weight changes

Underweight

Loss of weight is a common non-specific symptom of much serious mental and physical disease, normally one symptom among many. There is, however, one group of conditions collectively labelled 'anorexia nervosa' in which loss of weight resulting from self-starvation is the focus of concern. The patient refuses to eat, even if hungry, or eats only a little protein food but avoids carbohydrate and fat, secretly vomits after eating, takes purges and diuretics, or exercises to excess in an attempt to lose weight. Such patients have fears of being too fat, or of gaining weight, or of developing a sexually mature figure and are determined to stay thin to the point of endangering their lives. Anorexics are quite prepared to give false reports of weight gain and lie about themselves to allay concern about their condition. In adolescent girls and young women anorexia nervosa is accompanied by amenorrhoea and other effects of starvation. But refusal to eat an adequate amount of food does also occur, though much less often, in adolescent boys and in older women and men. There is frequently a disturbed relationship with a family member, usually a parent. Refusal to eat may be used to punish another or to attract special concern.

Since extreme weight loss predisposes to pneumonia, to gastric dilatation, and the patient dying of self-starvation, re-feeding is urgent. It must be carried out away from family pressures, in hospital and without home leave. Nurses who are firm, friendly, and aware of the deceptions such patients may practice can produce weight gain with the help of food supplements alone. Sometimes drugs are necessary to assist psychological treatment. Chlorpromazine (150–300 mg daily) stimulates appetite and causes weight gain. Amitriptyline is occasionally prescribed in the belief that there is an atypical depressive illness to be treated; amitriptyline, like chlorpromazine, has appetite-stimulating and weight-gaining effects over a period.

Bulimia nervosa, characterised by a morbid fear of becoming fat, irresistible urges to overeat followed by self-induced vomiting, purging, exercising and other measures to prevent weight gain, is almost exclusively a disorder of women. More so than anorexia nervosa, bulimia may affect older women and some who are married with children. Drugs, apart from tricyclic antidepressants for depression when present, have little part to play in treatment, which is based on cognitive therapy or various forms of psychotherapy.

Overweight

The psychiatrist encounters overweight as a result of long-term medication with phenothiazines, depot neuroleptics, tricyclic antidepressants, and lithium. Occasionally, an affective illness results in weight gain instead of loss, and an anxiety state causes ‘comfort’ overeating. Rarely, refractory obesity, thought to be ‘psychological’ after defying medical and surgical effort, is referred.

Obesity induced by psychotropic drugs nearly always disappears a few weeks after the drug is stopped. But stopping the drug may be inadvisable because of the risk of relapse. For lithium, a reduction in the daily dose may be tried, risking relapse for a slimmer figure, or carbamazepine, which does not seem to cause weight gain, substituted. A slimming diet may help, preferably with the advice of a dietician. Often, however, obesity is the price of drug control of positive symptoms of a psychosis, contributing to the characteristic clinical picture of the long-term patient. Obesity resulting from a depressive illness almost always disappears after successful treatment.

The treatment of gross obesity with a suspected psychological cause should be approached by investigating for evidence of overeating induced by anxiety, neurotic depression, or disturbed interpersonal relations. Treatment directed at these conditions, including the appropriate psychotropic drugs, sometimes reduces weight.

Appetite-suppressing drugs, phentermine, diethylpropion and mazindol, which are central stimulants related to amphetamine, are potentially addictive and therefore best avoided. Fenfluramine, a serotonin releaser with a sedative action and less addictive, can be prescribed in severe obesity. A two-month trial might result in a loss of 8 kg, after which the lost weight is often regained unless the treatment plan includes firmly planned dietary restriction. Psychotropic drugs have no place in the treatment of chronic obesity. A behavioural approach or a group like "Weight Watchers", which encourages reducing food intake and increasing energy output over the long term, can be successful.

Special weighing

It is worth knowing that total starvation will not produce a daily weight loss of more than 500 g in a sedentary person receiving water only; and that excessive feeding will not add more than a maximum of 200 g a day to the body's fat and flesh weight. Larger changes over 24 hours are due to losses or gains of body fluid (losses through urine, sweat or diarrhoea, perhaps). Emptying the bladder of overnight urine, volume 600 ml, means a weight loss of 600 g. Eating dinner will immediately add 500 g to body weight, drinks apart (these are rough values).

Weighing someone several times a day can be a check on whether an anorexic or bulimic patient has been eating normally or not. In patients prone to excessive water drinking (polydipsia, leading to water intoxication) comparison of the body weight at midday and at 4 p.m. with that at 8 a.m. may reveal the extent of overdrinking and the approach to the danger zone of hyponatraemia (below 120 mmol/l). A weight gain of 7% on the early morning body weight is the permitted maximum. In the rare Prader–Willi syndrome (obesity, poor growth, failure of sexual maturation, mental retardation) where the child or adolescent will rob refrigerators and break down doors to get food, frequent weighing can be used to detect the food intake and monitor the effect of treatment.

20 Lithium

Principally used to treat affective disorders and especially to prevent their recurrence, lithium salts also sometimes suppress schizophrenic symptoms and some states of aggression of uncertain diagnosis, including those in the mentally handicapped; they may also aid in preventing relapse of alcoholism, but this requires further study.

Lithium is widely used in psychiatry and, unusually for a psychotropic drug, considerable knowledge of its physiology has been obtained. As this has a direct bearing on its clinical use, an extensive account is given here.

Lithium is an element closely related to sodium and potassium (group 1 of the Periodic Table of elements) and like them is found widely distributed as salts in nature, in rocks, spa waters, and in the fluids of plants and animals. Traces are normal in the human body (about one-thousandth of the therapeutic level), and the lithium ion is distributed fairly evenly throughout the body water, intracellular and extracellular. Sodium in contrast is mostly extracellular and potassium intracellular.

Lithium has an immense number of actions in plants and animals, modifying the development of some, endocrine functions in others, and enzyme activities in a wide range of systems, but these activities all depend on particular concentrations of lithium ions. At the dilution present in normal untreated man, or resulting from drinking spa water, lithium can have no clinical effect. Most of the biochemical and biological actions of lithium described from the laboratory on isolated enzymes or organisms in experiments require lithium in 10 to 100 times the concentration achieved in therapy, way beyond the toxic limit in man. Therapeutic, human biochemical changes, and then toxic effects appear in a rather narrow range of concentrations, so that the safe, successful use of lithium in psychiatry depends on close control of the amount of lithium circulating in the blood. Understanding how this can vary is essential.

The lithium ion diffuses rapidly, so that it is absorbed from the stomach into the blood and enters most tissues; it soon begins to appear in the urine. It also appears in sweat but not, unless there is diarrhoea or failure of the lithium tablet to disintegrate, in the faeces. Lithium is not significantly stored anywhere in the body and, therefore, the amount circulating in the blood at any time depends only on the balance between the rate of intake by mouth and of excretion in the urine. There is usually both a rapid rate of absorption and a rapid excretion, provided renal function is normal. Lithium is excreted by glomerular filtration, with some reabsorption from the proximal tubule, as for sodium but much less efficiently. Renal blood flow, as decided by blood pressure, degree of vasoconstriction, hydration, and sodium intake, is therefore important. A diet low in sodium, heavy sweating as in hot weather or pyrexia, and hypotension from any cause, decrease urinary lithium and raise it in the blood, on constant oral dosing.

When a tablet of lithium citrate or carbonate is swallowed, providing it disintegrates and dissolves, the lithium concentration in the blood plasma rises rapidly to a sharp peak in one to four hours and then falls again, at first steeply and then more gently, in an exponential curve, as the lithium diffuses into the tissues or is lost in the urine (Fig. 2). The gentle fall, relatively flattening out, takes six to ten hours to reach the starting level, the time depending on the efficiency of renal excretion only. If lithium is taken thrice daily at, say, 8 a.m., 1 p.m. and 6 p.m., the second dose builds on top of the first, and the third on that to produce a very high peak before the fall, which will then last about 9–12 hours in most people. So the blood concentration is swinging between a very high level for a short time, and much lower levels for a considerable time, and is always changing. This has two important practical consequences.

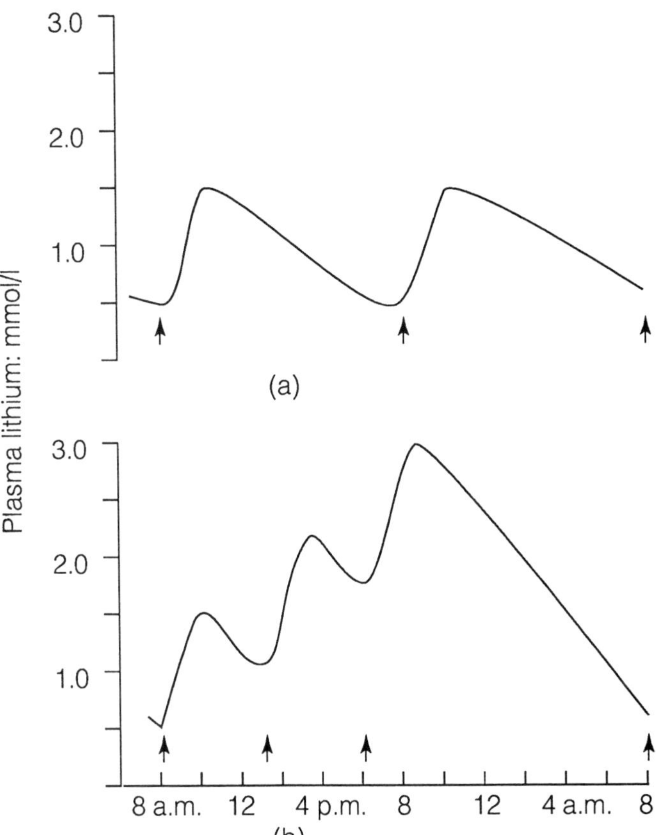

Fig. 2. Plasma lithium changes over hours after doses, indicated by arrows: (a) 12-hourly doses, (b) doses three times a day, at 8 a.m., 1 p.m. and 6 p.m.

(a) Unpleasant side-effects such as vomiting and diarrhoea, or polydipsia, are produced only by high levels. Therefore, keep the peaks down.

(b) It is essential to note the time when a blood sample for lithium measurement is taken, and the time when the last dose was taken also. Otherwise, the lithium value obtained by the laboratory cannot be correctly interpreted. To guide treatment the lithium is measured only when it is rather slowly changing, near the latter part of its fall. So the blood should be taken at least eight hours after the last dose, or just before taking the first dose of the day, if this is more convenient. This gives the minimum concentration of plasma lithium that is being reached on that dose schedule, and treatment is guided by these minima, and not by the heights reached from time to time. On the other hand, side-effects such as polyuria, obesity, vomiting, and toxic signs (see below) depend on the heights. Since there is no diurnal variation in lithium excretion, where more than one dose is given in the 24 hours the doses should be equally spaced (e.g. two, 12 hours apart, or three 8 hours apart). This will prevent a big peak at one part of the day while providing a satisfactory basal lithium level. Giving lithium thrice daily at four-hourly intervals may create a big peak in the late afternoon or early evening with diarrhoea, vomiting or nausea, or tremor. Another way of avoiding peaks is to prescribe sustained-release tablets, which let out their lithium more slowly than ordinary tablets and so spread out and soften the peak time. But it may still be necessary to give them 12-hourly, or more often, to split a big daily dose.

As dose follows dose, the 40 litres or so of body water become permeated by lithium ions in increasing amount until the urinary excretion rate equals the lithium intake. The basal plasma level and body water concentration of lithium then cease to rise, and this steady state will persist for very long periods as long as the daily dose remains constant and the individual remains in health and continues to live the same regular life, eating and drinking and exercising to similar extent. Pregnancy, an intercurrent infection, anaesthesia, or surgery will change the steady state and, therefore, demand new blood tests and possibly dose change. They do not mean that lithium must be stopped, but that closer control is needed. But once a steady state is achieved there is not the same need for frequent testing that there is when beginning treatment. Provided there is no life change, once in three or six months will be enough.

Poor renal function, as in the elderly or those with kidney disease (or even on regular renal dialysis) is not a contraindication to the use of lithium but means more care in choosing the daily dose and more frequent monitoring of the lithium by blood tests. Congestive cardiac failure, with fluctuating renal function and excess variable body water, perhaps with signs of oedema, is unlikely to be suitable for lithium because of the difficulty in establishing and keeping control. But the vast majority of patients to be put on lithium are physically healthy.

It is not known by what mechanism, or probably mechanisms, lithium produces its many neurological and psychiatric effects. Some side-effects occur quickly, and diarrhoea and some vomiting may result from direct local tissue action. But most effects, therapeutic or otherwise, take some days to begin to appear because lithium build-up in the brain is slower than in other tissues and some of its actions involve metabolic responses.

The division into quick and slow responses is important in recognising toxic overdosage. Acute overdose, raising the basal or minimum plasma level over 2.0 mmol/l, produces vomiting, which is likely to stop the taking of further lithium. If this happens, a blood sample should always be taken at once to confirm plasma level, because there are many causes of vomiting, for example food poisoning or cholecystitis. Recovery from too much lithium is quick if doses are stopped. In chronic overdose, however, where the plasma level creeps up from day to day, its slow rise does not provoke vomiting or nausea and is unrecognised until mental and neurological symptoms are evident. There is increasing clumsiness, ataxia, dysarthria, incoordination, vagueness, apathy, poor memory, disorientation; this may be noticed more by a relative than by the patient. If it is noticed within a week it can be reversed when lithium is stopped and its excretion promoted. Otherwise the condition progresses to coma and death, with plasma levels at 4–6 mmol/l.

Patients and relatives should always be instructed about the physiology of lithium, to know that regular eating and drinking are important, salt intake must be kept up and no special diets taken without medical agreement, to seek serum lithium checks in every physical illness and be taught the signs of chronic toxicity. Lithium is not addictive, quickly disappears when doses are missed and, in normal use, produces no symptoms of any sort in many patients. At the start, there may be a slight thirst and mild nocturia, which soon disappear. Tremor of the hands may appear at higher dose levels and high levels predispose to obesity or the sudden onset, after a few weeks, of thirst and polyuria (up to 5 litres a day). These effects are reversible by lithium readjustment.

Note that the plasma concentrations advised for success in therapy have been obtained by study of groups of American and British patients. The values might prove to be slightly different in other races or cultures. Also the therapeutic range is the range for the group studied as a whole. Thus, for mania, a plasma lithium level of 0.8–1.4 mmol/l is proposed. This means that no one was found to improve at less than 0.8 mmol/l and that taking the level above 1.4 mmol/l did not result in improvement of anyone who had not yet responded. But a given individual may not respond at 1.0, yet do so at 1.2, while another may have recovered on 0.8. So when a suitable patient does not respond at the lower lithium level, increase it, if necessary to the top of the range, before concluding the individual is non-responsive.

Uses

Lithium (Camcolit, Phasal, Priadel, Liskonum, Litarex) may be used for:

(a) treatment of hypomania
(b) prevention of recurrent depression and mania, or lessening of distressing cyclothymia
(c) treatment of irritability and aggression in the mentally handicapped
(d) drug combination treatments of depression or schizophrenia.

Treatment of hypomania and aggression

Because it is slow to act, lithium is not the treatment of choice in manic illness, where a neuroleptic will be preferred. But is has some value in hypomanic cases, especially out-patients, because it is easy and safe to handle, and should show results within a week.

Start with 1200–1600 mg (30–40 mmol) lithium carbonate in daily divided as doses at 8 a.m. and 8 p.m., or 8 a.m., 4 p.m., midnight (smaller daily intake for the elderly, or those with poor kidney function), and take a *timed* blood sample (see above) at five days, and three days for the elderly. Then change oral dose to adjust plasma level to the desired value, above 0.8 and below 1.4 mmol/l lithium. Doses can be altered every week when monitoring with blood tests. Once it is clear the right plasma level has been reached, confirm its stability on the same dose by two-monthly blood tests, and then it will suffice to test the patient three-monthly or even half-yearly.

Young patients may need and tolerate up to 2400 mg daily. The same procedure is appropriate for the aggressive mentally handicapped.

Notes

(a) Look out for missed doses by asking patient, relatives and staff, and by inspecting the medicine bottle. They upset the steady state and spoil control, with dangerous possibilities. The patients should be warned of these to help them to confess irregularity and strive towards complete dosage.

(b) Side-effects will be less if lithium is not taken as one daily dose but split into two or three equally spaced doses.

(c) Hand tremor, worse on voluntary movement, is the most troublesome side-effect in ordinary treatment. It may be avoided by rearranging the dose schedule to keep the plasma peaks down (see above) or giving 30–60 mg propranolol daily in divided doses.

Prophylactic treatment of recurrent illness and other uses

In prophylaxis the effective plasma level is lower (0.5–0.8 mmol/l) although, occasionally, a level of 1.0 mmol/l or higher may be necessary. A daily intake of 800 mg lithium carbonate will be enough for most people. Again, adjust doses weekly to the desired stable plasma level and, provided circumstances do not change, six-monthly follow-up tests will suffice. Make sure the patient understands about physiology and toxic signs.

When should one consider prophylaxis? One does not want someone to embark on long-term drug taking without good reason. Affective disorders recur. If two or more attacks come within three years, recurrence is likely to be frequent and worth preventing. But do not start lithium after a first attack of illness, when the next attack, if at all, may be years away. Very mild attacks may suggest postponing prophylaxis but the more dangerous the attack is, for example high suicidal risk or disastrous social effects, the sooner one will want to try prevention.

If lithium is effective in prevention it will need to be continued indefinitely. Ten years without relapse is no guarantee of future health if lithium is then stopped. If it is stopped it must be by gradual reduction, because there is a risk of a new manic attack almost at once after sudden withdrawal. Rapid bipolar cyclers (4–6 attacks in the year) do not usually do very well with lithium prophylaxis and carbamazepine may be better. Where both alone have failed, combining the two may succeed.

In the treatment of depressive illness, where a tricyclic such as imipramine has failed, the addition of lithium carbonate, 800 mg or more per day, may result in early improvement. In the treatment of schizophrenia, the addition of lithium in the same way to a neuroleptic may bring better results. These helpful drug combinations are still a matter of experiment and study, and no plasma level ranges have been established.

Preparation of the patient

The ordinary physically healthy person requires no physical preparation beyond the routine taking of medical history and physical examination. In the past all kinds of fears of the dangers of lithium have been expressed, based on theories or incomplete observations. In particular it was thought at one time that lithium did significant renal damage, because it was seen to do so under some circumstances in rats, because human renal biopsy showed some histological changes, and because lithium can produce nephrogenic diabetes insipidus, in which the kidney becomes reversibly insensitive to antidiuretic hormone because of a specific enzyme inhibition. But extensive follow-up of many lithium-treated patients has not shown any development of renal disease or increased mortality, nor changes in sensitive tests of renal function.

As for ability to excrete lithium in urine, this is best judged by the excretion of lithium as shown by the fall in plasma lithium level with time after successive doses, rather than by such crude tests of renal function as creatinine clearance or blood urea. If one has the slightest suspicion that a patient (e.g. an elderly person) may not have good renal function, start lithium very cautiously, 400 mg daily say, and determine the plasma concentration at two or five days thereafter, adjusting dose as before to reach therapeutic levels.

Another fear has been the development of hypothyroidism, which may occur very early in treatment or only after years, and is as likely on low as on high doses. It comes on suddenly, without warning from routine function tests, and is recognised clinically by slowing, vague depression, intolerance of cold – it is therefore difficult to distinguish from the onset of a depressive phase. This is where the laboratory tests become very valuable. If hypothyroidism is present, it responds to thyroxine and lithium can be continued. If lithium is withdrawn, the thyroid will probably recover in about two months.

Routine tests of renal, thyroid and cardiac function before commencing lithium in the absence of clinical evidence of disease and then every three to four months thereafter have become common practice. The grounds for this derive in part from medico-legal reasons. These are no substitute for the doctor clinically assessing patients in a thorough manner when seen, looking for any sensitivity to the drug, including toxic side-effects and, if present, trying to relate them to the dose schedule. When tests are done regularly, a foolproof system of noting and filing results must be devised. Too often, results go astray or float loosely in the case notes.

Lithium can modify the electrocardiogram but there is no evidence that, as used in psychiatry, it has a deleterious effect on function. Lithium can also enter bone in place of calcium. However, there are no pathological fractures to report in chronic lithium takers, nor any radiographic evidence of increasing osteoporosis. Doing a battery of cardiac, renal, and endocrine tests is therefore inessential, unless one fears that clinically one will miss some occult disease, or is frightened at the possibility of a legal case if treatment fails.

For physically ill people the matter is quite different, and a physician's opinion can be helpful in judging the extent of pathology. Also, lithium does not mix with some of the drugs in medical use. Thiazide diuretics and non-steroidal anti-inflammatory anti-arthritic drugs, such as indomethacin, and piroxicam, diminish excretion of lithium in urine and may raise the plasma level to become toxic. Tetracycline is also to be avoided or treated with circumspection. Two skin diseases, psoriasis and acne, may be made worse by lithium.

Side-effects

Early

Vomiting within minutes of swallowing a dose usually results from gastric irritation and can be avoided by taking the tablets with milk.

Vomiting four to eight hours after a dose can be due to a high plasma lithium level affecting the brain-stem; diarrhoea at the same time is due to high lithium levels, probably acting directly on the gut nerve net.

A mild degree of thirst, dry feeling and lessened feeling of concentration have also been reported.

There may be tremor of hands, and clumsy fingers.

Late

Polydipsia, diabetes insipidus (nephrogenic), obesity, and hypothyroidism may occur.

The chief drug interactions of practical importance are described above (pp. 136, 138).

Toxic signs

These are increasing clumsiness, incoordination, ataxia, slurred speech, and vagueness, impaired memory, sluggish thinking, disorientation. Distinguish this picture from returning depression, from neurological disease, and acute brain syndrome from other causes. The condition becomes more marked, leading to coma and death if untreated reasonably soon.

Effects on foetus and infant

During the first three months of pregnancy, when the foetus is being formed, there is a small risk of lithium producing cardiac malformations. Congenital anomalies appear quite often in the newborn who have not been subject to any drugs. Deciding whether to stop a pregnant woman's prophylactic lithium for the first trimester of pregnancy is a matter of balancing the risks to her, and to successful conclusion of the pregnancy if she has a relapse into mania or depression at this time, against the risk to the baby of birth defect.

A foetus exposed to lithium in late pregnancy may be born with hypotonia and hypothyroidism, but these should clear soon. A newborn infant getting breast milk from a mother taking lithium will be receiving a lithium dose which the infantile kidney has difficulty in excreting. Lithium can easily be measured in breast milk and will be higher in a woman on a high basal plasma level of lithium. Hypothyroidism and goitre is the main risk to the baby; it might be less with low maternal plasma lithium, or where breast feeds are supplemented by other milk. Again, the pros and cons of breast feeding in the individual case must be considered.

Preparations

When prescribing, whether citrate or carbonate is to be preferred is uncertain. No injectable form is available. Liquid for oral administration can be prepared from lithium chloride or citrate.

Lithium carbonate (100 mg is 2.7 mmol Li) –
- tablets: 250 mg, 400 mg (Camcolit)
- controlled-release tablets: 300 mg (Phasal), 200 mg, 400 mg (Priadel), 450 mg (Liskonum)

Lithium citrate –
- controlled-release tablets: 564 mg (6 mmol Li) (Litarex)

21 Tricyclic antidepressants

Amitriptyline and imipramine are the two oldest and best-known drugs for treating depressive illness. Their chemical structure, three joined rings of atoms with a centrally attached tail or side-chain on one side, is termed 'tricyclic' (Fig. 3). The central ring has seven atoms, not six as in phenothiazines, a structure which makes the molecule 'V'-shaped and unable to lie flat. The tricyclic central ring structure makes the drug antidepressant: the side-chain influences potency and sedative action. Tricyclics are not only antidepressants: cyproheptadine (Periactin) is used as an appetite stimulant, carbamazepine (Tegretol) as an anticonvulsant, as well as an antimanic and a prophylactic against bipolar affective illness.

The wide range of tricyclics to choose from is the result of minor structural modifications of the fundamental molecular ground plan, achieved by drug company research for commercial as well as scientific reasons. They are called 'tricyclics' simply because their molecules are made essentially of three linked rings of atoms. If a fourth ring is added, for instance at right angles to the other three, as in maprotiline or mianserin, then the compound can be called tetracyclic but is still essentially one of the same clinical pharmacological group. There is little established basis for preferring one structural variation to another. Imipramine and amitriptyline have been firmly established as superior to placebo but newer drugs often have not. New antidepressants have to be proved to be as good as these two and have advantages such as fewer side-effects in therapeutic dosage or lower cost before being preferred. In general, use a new drug only if the patient has an idiosyncratic reaction to an old and proved one. If one

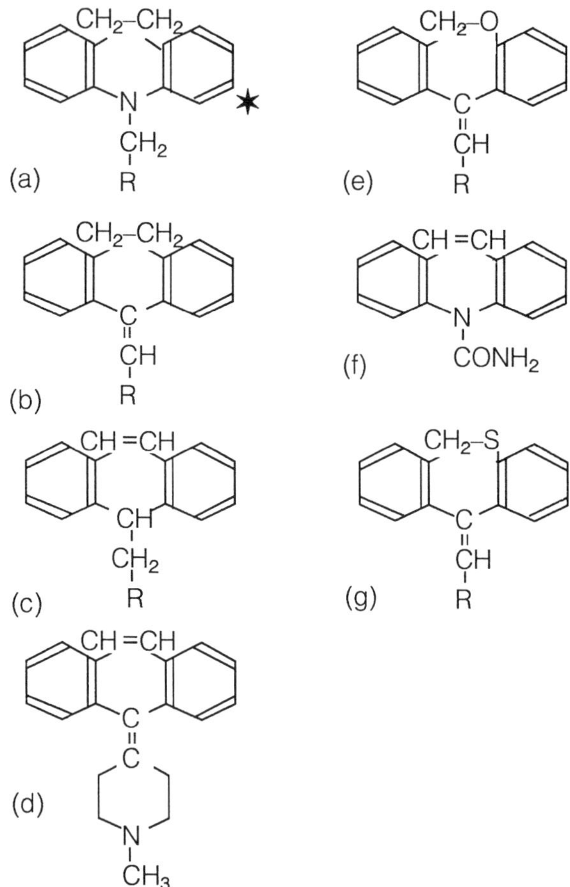

*Fig. 3. Tricyclic drug structures. (a) For imipramine, R is $-CH_2CH_2N(CH_3)_2$; for desipramine R is $-CH_2CH_2N(CH_3)H$; for trimipramine R is $-CH(CH_3)-CH_2N(CH_3)_2$; when a chlorine atom instead of a hydrogen atom is attached to the carbon marked * in the imipramine structure, clomipramine is formed. (b) For amitriptyline, R is as for imipramine; for nortriptyline, R is as for desipramine. (c) For protriptyline, R is as for desipramine. (d) Cyproheptadine, (e) doxepin, (f) carbamazepine, and (g) dothiepin (in e and g R is as in imipramine)*

tricyclic fails after an adequate trial another is unlikely to do better therapeutically. But where a tricyclic, though working, produces troublesome side-effects, a change to another active drug may avoid this problem.

All tricyclics are slow to act therapeutically – between one and three weeks. In contrast, side-effects (due to anticholinergic properties) are quick to appear – dry mouth, visual disturbance, postural hypotension, sweating, and constipation may be evident after 24 hours. Amitriptyline and also, to a lesser extent, imipramine cause drowsiness, which may be put to use for night sedation. Nortriptyline and desipramine, derived from them by a slight alteration at the tip of the side-chain, are not sedative. Within a few days these side-effects lessen and usually disappear. Claims that newer drugs produce fewer side-effects are often based only on smaller doses being used, and this often means less clinical potency, offset perhaps by the psychological benefit of taking something new. But some do have less anticholinergic effect.

Tricyclics can cause serious reactions, particularly in the physically ill. They cause: acute retention of urine in the elderly, particularly men with large prostates; acute glaucoma in those with narrow-angle glaucoma; tachycardia, arrhythmia and heart block in those with already damaged hearts. They interfere with the control of high blood pressure by adrenergic-blocking drugs (e.g. guanethidine), which act by preventing noradrenaline release and uptake; and they potentiate the action of adrenaline in local anaesthetics by preventing adrenalin re-uptake, thereby causing a rise in blood pressure. They may cause fits in those predisposed to epileptic attacks. A withdrawal reaction – nausea, vomiting, sweating, insomnia – sometimes occurs on sudden withdrawal of the drug.

The blood levels of some tricyclics can now be measured. These levels are total values which comprise a small pharmacologically active fraction dissolved free in the water of the plasma plus a large pharmacologically inactive fraction bound to the plasma protein. This needs to be borne in mind. Upon metabolism amitriptyline quickly gives rise to nortriptyline, and imipramine, likewise, to desipramine;

thereafter, hydroxylation occurs at either of two places, on a carbon of the central ring (clinically active) or on a side ring (inactive). Withdrawal of drug and metabolites from the tissues, and excretion, is rapid. Excretion is chiefly in the urine.

Overdose of imipramine or amitriptyline leads in one to five hours to unconsciousness, with a catastrophic fall in blood pressure, cardiac arrythmias, epileptic fits, and sometimes status epilepticus. Stomach washout, control of fits, and maintenance of blood pressure, and hence of kidney function, must be carried out in a medical ward under specialist guidance. Prognosis is good where treatment begins shortly after the overdose.

Amitriptyline is described in detail as the typical tricyclic drug. This does not mean we regard it as pre-eminent – we could equally well have placed imipramine, for instance, in this position. To avoid tiresome repetition of shared properties, other tricyclics are only briefly treated or listed. They vary in their sedating and anticholinergic properties, and this may influence choice.

The commonest cause of failure to relieve depressive illness with a drug is to use too small a dose. As long as side-effects are small the dose can be raised. A second cause is impatience: at least two weeks' action is needed.

Amitriptyline

Amitriptyline (Tryptizol, Lentizol) may be used for:

(a) depressive illness, especially with 'biological' symptoms
(b) panic reactions and phobias
(c) nocturnal enuresis in children.

For adults, start with oral tablets after food, 25 mg thrice daily, or simply 50–100 mg at night since then a separate hypnotic may not be needed and morning anxiety and agitation will be better controlled. After two days the dose can be raised, and raised again as required. A daily intake of 150 mg is quite usual. There will be no response for at least two weeks, and some patients will need to go to 300 mg daily to improve. Individuals differ in their tolerance of side-effects but it usually increases in a few days, which is the reason for starting with low doses and raising by steps. If side-effects continue to be a problem, try a different tricyclic. Where agitation and insomnia remain poorly controlled, small doses of a phenothiazine such as thioridazine, or a benzodiazepine such as diazepam, may be a helpful addition.

Adults who complain of indigestion or vomiting with tablets may try syrup instead. Intramuscular injections guarantee medication and are psychologically impressive, so may have an additional powerful placebo effect. Slow-release preparations probably have no advantage over tablets in similar dose and may be more expensive.

Antidepressants must be continued for some time after recovery. For how long is uncertain. For a first illness four weeks after recovery may be a reasonable time, then reduce the dose in steps. If depressive symptoms begin to return, go back to the original higher dose and try reduction again in another four weeks. Do not be in a hurry to stop treatment. After a third attack in three years prophylaxis by continuing the tricyclic is a reasonable line of treatment, but the drug must be continued at the dose level found therapeutic and not reduced. Alternatively, lithium or carbamazepine may be given (q.v.). The decision when to start prophylaxis, and when to stop it, depends on weighing the social consequences of a further depression, its likely severity, the risk of suicide, the side-effects of the drug, and the patient's motivations.

A similar approach is used for panic reactions and phobias, and in these even low initial doses can lessen anxiety quickly.

In children amitriptyline (25 or 50 mg at night) reduces frequency of bed-wetting. It is less effective and more upsetting than an electric alarm and should not be used where incontinence has physical illness as its cause (see "Disorders of childhood", p. 94).

Brain damage in children and in adults is no contraindication to tricyclic treatment, and depression after a stroke can respond well to the drug. Heart damage, however, in particular myocardial infarction, carries some risk of dysrhythmia with a tricyclic, and electroconvulsive therapy (ECT) at 12 weeks or more from the attack may be safer. Tricyclics in therapeutic dose are not toxic to the healthy heart and may even have some anti-arrhythmic properties. Stabilised treatment for hypertension may be upset. Elderly men with enlarged prostates may get urinary retention; and glaucoma can be made worse, with pain in the eye from increased intraocular pressure so that, before starting treatment, the advice of an ophthalmologist is desirable.

Side-effects

These are quick (within hours) or slow (after two weeks or more of treatment). The quick are very common: drowsiness, oversedation, indigestion, dry mouth, constipation, blurring of vision, headache, dizziness, postural hypotension and difficulty in urination. The slow, in order of increasing rarity, are: weight gain (lost again when drug is stopped), shaking of limbs, hypomania, grand mal attack, toxic hallucinosis (like that from benzhexol), paralytic ileus causing acute abdominal pain, and Parkinsonian tremor with facial immobility and stiff movements. The last is more likely when lithium also is taken, and is an interactive effect.

Patients on monoamine oxidase inhibitor (MAOI) drugs or who have taken them in the previous seven days run the risk, when given amitriptyline (or another amine tricyclic), of developing a severe vascular headache with high blood pressure. Treat this with phentolamine (5–10 mg i.v.). But combined MAOI/tricyclic therapy for resistant depression is possible (see p. 156). Hyperpyrexia is less common.

Note that some phenothiazine drugs given concurrently with a tricyclic inhibit its metabolism and raise its blood level in consequence.

Preparations

Tablets: 10, 25, 50 mg
Capsules: 75 mg
Sustained-release capsules (Lentizol): 25, 50, 75 mg
Syrup: 10 mg per 5 ml
Injection: ampoule of 10 ml contains 10 mg/ml

Nortriptyline

The clinical effects are like those of amitriptyline except that nortriptyline (Allegron, Aventyl) has little sedative or hypnotic action. In fact, nortriptyline is rapidly produced in the body from amitriptyline so it is not surprising that the two are almost indistinguishable. Doses can, however be a little lower – 75 mg daily may be enough, producing a plasma concentration of 50–150 ng/ml or about 200–600 nmol/l.

Preparations

Tablets: 10, 25 mg
Capsules: 10, 25 mg
Liquid: 10 mg/5 ml

Imipramine, desipramine, trimipramine, lofepramine

Very like amitriptyline in all respects, imipramine (Tofranil) can be used in the same way in the same doses, up to 300 mg daily. Desipramine is the *counterpart* of nortriptyline, in this case being the metabolite of imipramine, but is rather expensive. Trimipramine differs by one carbon atom in the side-chain from imipramine and appears to have very similar properties. Lofepramine also belongs to this group of drugs, and metabolises to desipramine.

Preparations

Imipramine –
tablets: 10, 25 mg
syrup: 25 mg/5 ml
Desipramine –
tablets: 25 mg (Pertofran) (up to 200 mg daily)
Trimipramine –
tablets: 10, 25 mg (Surmontil) (up to 300 mg daily)
capsules: 50 mg
Lofepramine –
tablets: 70 mg (Gamanil) (up to 210 mg daily)

Clomipramine

Clomipramine (Anafranil) is imipramine with one chlorine atom added to a side ring, and some people consider it made more potent weight-for-weight thereby. It is used for depressive illnesses in general, but has also been recommended for depressions resistant to ordinary treatments, in daily dose of 150 mg combined with 2–3 g tryptophan daily and lithium carbonate to produce a plasma level of 0.5–0.8 mmol/l Li (tryptophan has now been withdrawn).

It has also been used with good effect in obsessional and phobic illness, even without accompanying depression (high-dose imipramine may also be effective here), but particularly when given by slow intravenous infusion, the only imipramine group preparation suitable for this method. On day 1, 25 or 50 mg drug in 500 ml saline or 5% dextrose is given over two hours, with pulse and blood pressure records before, half-hourly, during and for two hours afterwards. If there are no adverse effects, the dose is increased by 25 mg each successive day to a maximum of 250 mg, and it may be possible to decrease the fluid volume and speed the infusion somewhat. Usually the infusion is given on five days of each seven, the remaining two days substituting oral doses, and the treatment continued for two to three weeks. If symptoms remit, oral clomipramine may be continued. Note that the treatment is not very suitable for patients with liver damage or cardiac conditions, and can produce all the tricyclic side-effects in severe form; in addition there is a risk of venous thrombosis (pain), ataxia and vertigo, impotence, and haematuria.

Preparations

Capsules: 10, 25, 50 mg
Sustained-release tablet: 75 mg
Syrup: 25 mg/5 ml
Injection: 2 ml ampoule contains 25 mg.

Dothiepin

Dothiepin (Prothiaden) resembles amitriptyline in its sedative and antidepressant effect, but is much less potent, so that a minimum of 100 mg daily must be given to have more than a placebo effect. It is said to have milder side-effects and to be particularly suitable for the elderly.

Preparations

Tablets: 75 mg
Capsules: 25 mg.

Mianserin

For depressive illness, especially retarded depressions, in divided daily doses of 30–90 mg, the merit of mianserin

(Bolvidon, Norval) is to have no cardiac effects, not to interfere with antihypertensive treatment or be anticholinergic and hence is useful in the elderly. On the other hand, it can cause great drowsiness (hence introduce the drug gradually in ascending dose), and epilepsy and aplastic anaemia have been reported so that a monthly blood examination is advised for the first three months of treatment. Agranulocytosis (possibly with sore throat or fever) is a particular risk in the elderly.

Preparations

Tablets: 10, 20, 30 mg.

Fluoxetine

This newly introduced antidepressant (Prozac) is said to act selectively by inhibiting the reuptake of serotonin by pre-synaptic nerve terminals. It is rapidly absorbed and metabolised, mainly in the liver. The drug has a long half-life and therefore wait three weeks after giving it up, before starting an MAOI; the dosage is 20 mg daily. Compared with the older tricyclic drugs, it has fewer anticholinergic effects and is less sedative. It may cause weight loss.

Preparations

Capsules: 20 mg.

Carbamazepine

Carbamazepine (Tegretol), a close relation of imipramine, was originally introduced for epilepsy, and a full account of it is given on p. 206, under "Anti-epileptic drugs". It has also found use in the treatment of trigeminal neuralgia and, more recently, has proved valuable in the prevention of recurrent attacks of manic–depressive illness, especially short-cycle bipolar cases, and in the treatment of manic attacks. It is prone to interaction with other drugs; it has to be introduced gradually and the dose readjusted, as it induces its own destruction by the liver. Start with 100 mg twice daily in the first week and 200 mg twice daily in the second, expecting to level off at 600–1200 mg daily in divided doses, sometimes more (but see the account on p. 207).

Preparations

Tablets: 100, 200, 400 mg
Sustained-release tablets: 200, 400 mg
Liquid: 100 mg/5 ml, bottle contains 300 ml.

Related drugs

The maximum daily dose is given in parentheses in each case.

Protriptyline (Concordin), tablets: 5, 10 mg (60 mg).
Butriptyline (Evadyne), tablets: 25, 50 mg (150 mg).
Doxepin (Sinequan), capsules: 10, 25, 50, 75 mg (300 mg).
Maprotiline (Ludiomil), tablets: 10, 25, 50, 75 mg (150 mg).
Iprindole (Prondol), tablets: 15, 30 mg (180 mg).
Trazodone (Molipaxin), capsules: 50, 100 mg; tablets: 150 mg (300 mg).
Viloxazine (Vivalan), tablets: 50 mg (400 mg).
Fluvoxamine (Faverin), tablets: 50 mg (200 mg).
Amoxapine (Asendis), tablets: 25, 50, 100, 150 mg (300 mg).
Sertraline (Lustral), tablets: 50, 100 mg (150 mg).
Paroxetine (Seroxat): doses etc. unavailable at time of writing.

Drug combinations

These are given for information only: we do not recommend them.

Limbitrol-10: 25 mg amitriptyline with 10 mg of the chlordiazepoxide Librium (Limbitrol-5 is half-strength).
Motival: 10 mg nortriptyline plus 0.5 mg fluphenazine (Motipress is similar but three times stronger).
Triptafen: 25 mg amitriptyline plus 2 mg perphenazine Triptafen-M has 10 mg amitriptyline plus 2 mg perphenazine.

22 Monoamine oxidase inhibitors

The uses of monoamine oxidase inhibitors (MAOIs) in psychiatry do not fall into neat categories. They have been described as sedatives, euphoriants, antidepressants, and antiphobics. It is more rational, however, to think of them simply as having some slow central nervous modifying action, changing the balance of brain functions in some as yet unknown way: some patients are undoubtedly helped by MAOIs, some even specifically by one particular drug only of the group. The indications are atypical depressions and where tricyclic antidepressants have failed (see p. 68).

Most MAOIs are hydrazine derivatives and contain the chemical grouping -NH-NH- in the side-chain, exposed, as in phenelzine, or embedded, as in isocarboxazid. Hydrazines are inactivated by acetylation in the liver, by which -NH-NH- is converted to -NH-NH-CO-CH_3. Speed of acetylation is genetically determined, some individuals being fast and others slow acetylators.

The non-hydrazine derivatives are amphetamine and more particularly its relative tranylcypromine (Parnate). They may be classified by clinical usage in this section of the pharmacopoeia, although by chemistry and metabolism they are distinct. They have some MAOI activity, but are considered separately in the next chapter.

The MAOI drugs combine irreversibly with and thus inactivate the enzymes that oxidise serotonin, tyramine and other amines. These amines may be neurotransmitters, potential toxins in foods, or ingredients of medicines. The enzymes inactivated are found in many parts of the body, for instance the intestinal wall, the platelets of the blood, the heart, liver, kidney and lung, and the brain. The enzymes in different tissues differ in the relative efficiency with which they oxidise different amines, and their relative sensitivities to different MAOI drugs also differ. Thus the MAO-A enzyme, which oxidises serotonin and noradrenaline, is inhibited by phenelzine, which is antidepressant. the MAO-B enzyme oxidises dopamine and is inhibited by selegiline (Eldepryl), used in Parkinsonism.

Apart from amine oxidases, the drugs inactivate other enzymes, particularly liver hydroxylases which metabolise barbiturates, anti-Parkinsonian drugs, tricyclic antidepressants or phenytoin and other organic chemicals. They may also inactivate pyridoxal, a co-enzyme derived from vitamin B_6 (pyridoxine), which plays a part in many processes in the metabolism of organic acids and of the neurotransmitter GABA. These inactivations are rapid whereas the clinical effects are slow, so it is difficult to know how the drugs act, and whether their inhibition of monoamine oxidases, simply one among several inhibitions, is what matters.

Enzymes are proteins which are continually being broken down and resynthesised during life. When an enzyme is irreversibly inhibited and hence functionally destroyed, fresh enzyme gradually resynthesised in the course of two or three weeks eventually replaces all that has been destroyed, unless fresh inhibitor is continually added. In treatment, free MAOI disappears by metabolism and excretion, leaving inactivated enzymes which take time to be replaced. This time for recovery is why it is advisable to wait a week or so after stopping an MAOI before starting another drug (e.g. a tricyclic), and also why measurement of an MAOI drug blood level may tell little about the degree of enzyme inhibition.

Because of the protean effects of MAOI, caution and watchfulness are required: caution in deciding to use them and to mix them with other drugs, and watchfulness for the physical signs of side-effects and of toxicity. They are frequently hypotensive, especially in causing postural hypotension, but paradoxically facilitate hypertensive episodes, sometimes with severe headache, particularly when tyramine-rich foods are eaten. Hence, patients should be advised not to eat any cheese, and to avoid pickled herrings, Marmite, etc. (see below). Alcohol is best avoided, especially heavy wines, but also non-alcoholic beers may cause problems. Bananas, except perhaps the skins, and broad beans, except the pods, are safe.

The MAOIs may cause ankle oedema and puffy hands because of fluid retention. They may be hypoglycaemic because they inhibit the decay of natural insulin. They have caused jaundice. They are unsafe combined with amphetamines or methyldopa; they prevent the metabolism and so enhance the effect of morphine and pethidine, and likewise of anti-Parkinsonian drugs, tricyclic antidepressants, barbiturates, and phenytoin. If an MAOI is added to the prescription of a patient already stabilised on one or more of these other drugs, the stability may be upset, and a toxic overdose develop. But the fact remains that, in spite of many potential risks, troubles are uncommon in practice when care is taken.

Patients often carry a card explaining they are taking an MAOI, so that other practitioners, including anaesthetists and dentists, may know and prescribe their drugs with appropriate caution to avoid unpleasant or dangerous interactions.

Phenelzine and isocarboxazid

Phenelzine (Nardil) and the related drug isocarboxazid (Marplan) may be used for:

(a) atypical depressive states
(b) depressions unresponsive to tricyclic drugs
(c) phobic anxiety states.

Start with 15 mg thrice daily and after one week increase to 60 mg daily if side-effects are not marked. Raise to 75 mg daily after a second week and so continue for at least two weeks. It is possible to give 90 mg daily. Elderly patients, as usual, will require lower doses than these. Antidepressant response is slow, taking two to six weeks.

Combination with tricyclics

Start the tricyclic antidepressant drug first in a low dose, for example 100 mg at night, or not more than 150 mg daily. Either amitriptyline or imipramine may be used. Then introduce MAOI drug, twice and then thrice daily in usual dose. Inquire carefully for side-effects after two or three days, at one, two and three weeks, and whenever the patient is seen thereafter. If the patient is already taking an MAOI it is possible to start a tricyclic with it by small doses at night, very slowly increasing.

Combination with lithium

Drug-resistant depression may respond to 15 mg phenelzine thrice daily, plus lithium carbonate to give plasma lithium 0.5–0.8 mmol/l. The drug has some sedative action and may quickly counteract insomnia in some states of tension.

Side-effects and interactions

The drug should not be given during infective hepatitis, obstructive jaundice, liver cirrhosis or congestive cardiac failure. Patients must be told to avoid all self-medication (for colds, etc., because of the risk of interactions with ephedrine), and should avoid meat or yeast extracts, pickled herrings, chicken liver, wine, cheeses in large quantity, or even in small, especially for American processed, Camembert, Brie, Stilton and Gorgonzola.

Common side-effects are sweating, dry mouth, weakness, and faintness, especially from postural hypotension. Less frequent are tingling paraesthesia in upper or lower limbs (for which pyridoxine, 50 mg daily, is sometimes given), ankle oedema, tremor. Toxic reactions include hyperpyrexia, convulsions, agitation and confusional states in which hallucinations may be prominent. Depressed patients are said sometimes to swing into hypomania because of the drug.

In cases of hypertensive crisis, give phentolamine (5–10 mg i.v.).

Because of drug interactions avoid sympatheticomimetic amines (amphetamine, fenfluramine, ephedrine), sometimes present in proprietary cold cures and cough medicines, antihypertensive drugs (such as methyldopa, guanethidine), and antihistamines. Note that preparations of local anaesthetic sometimes contain sympatheticomimetic amines. Sensitivity to insulin may be increased, perhaps by blocking insulin destruction, and hence increasing sensitivity to oral anti-diabetic drugs, resulting in unexpected hypoglycaemia. Morphine and pethidine are contraindicated, but not other analgesics. Metabolism of many drugs by the liver, for instance barbiturates and phenytoin, may be interfered with.

Preparations

Phenelzine –
  tablets: 15 mg
Isocarboxazid (Marplan) –
  tablets: 10 mg (30 mg maximum daily dose, otherwise use as for phenelzine).

Note

A new set of MAOI drugs, short-acting and reversible and with antidepressant activity, is on the way. Moclobemide is one such. Extended clinical experience is awaited.

23 Stimulants

Stimulants are a rather diverse group of drugs mostly related to amphetamine (which is why fenfluramine has been listed here, although it is an appetite suppressant rather than a stimulant).

Tranylcypromine

Although tranylcypromine (Parnate) has less marked MAOI action than phenelzine, it is strongly sympatheticomimetic and side-effects and interactions are similar. The same drugs and foods must be avoided, as hypertensive and other side-effects are not infrequent, but liver damage is less likely.

In a dose of 10 mg twice or thrice daily it is used against depressions where phenelzine might be prescribed. However, like amphetamine, to which it is chemically related, tranylcypromine has some *immediate* euphoriant effect and may cause insomnia, so is best taken in the morning. The immediate effect encourages the patient, but occasionally leads to dependence.

Preparations

Tablets: 10 mg.

Note. Under the name Parstelin is sold a combination of tranylcypromine (10 mg) and the phenothiazine drug trifluoperazine (Stelazine) (1 mg) which is used when sedation is required in addition to antidepressant activity. The evidence for the special value of Parstelin is limited: part of it is by analogy with amphetamine, the therapeutic effects of which are certainly helpfully modified by combination with amylobarbitone.

Dexamphetamine

Dexamphetamine (Dexedrine) may be used for:

(a) narcolepsy
(b) Kleine–Levin syndromes
(c) hyperkinetic children
(d) epilepsy, to increase alertness.

Amphetamines act as central stimulants and consequently have a variety of psychological effects. They are used, often illegally, for their euphoriant action and for counteracting fatigue or for suppressing appetite. Tolerance for these effects, *especially* the euphoriant effect, develops rapidly. There is therefore a serious risk of inducing dependence. For this reason, the prescription of amphetamine is controlled under Schedule 2 of the Misuse of Drugs Act. Theft of amphetamine occurs and sometimes patients sell their tablets.

To treat narcolepsy or Kleine–Levin syndrome start with 10 mg in the morning and increase in 10 mg steps each week until control is achieved or a maximum of 50 mg per day is reached. Clomipramine may be even more effective.

For children with hyperkinesis (see under "Disorders of childhood", p. 96) start with 2.5 mg in the morning and increase weekly in steps of 2.5 mg to a maximum of 20 mg daily, divided into two or three doses daily.

Dexamphetamine (5 mg two or three times a day) can reverse the drowsiness and inattention caused by anti-convulsant drugs.

Because of the risk of dependence, amphetamine should not be used as an appetite suppressant. Use fenfluramine (p. 161) if a drug must be prescribed.

The drug may cause insomnia, especially if taken late in the day.

Long-term use in high dosage may retard children's growth because of appetite suppression. Height and weight must therefore be monitored. High doses can cause perseveration of attention, with consequent learning problems, so concentration must also be monitored. Tics and stereotyped behaviour can be made worse and Tourette's syndrome unmasked.

Misery and tearfulness can appear, usually transiently, in children taking therapeutic doses. Large doses produce agitation, excitement and even a paranoid psychosis with hallucinations in adults. Tachycardia, palpitations and a rise in blood pressure can all occur, so heart rate and blood pressure need to be examined regularly.

Beware of increasing tolerance and the development of psychological dependence. A depressive mood swing on stopping can occur. Beware of parents ill-treating a child by giving excessive doses.

The drug should not be given to people with a history of cardiovascular disease, hypertension, tics or drug dependence. It causes hypertensive and hyperpyrexial reactions if given with a monoamine oxidase inhibitor (MAOI). Amphetamine antagonises the antihypertensive effect of guanethidine.

Preparations

Tablets: 5 mg.

Pemoline

Pemoline (Volital) is a stimulant, like methylphenidate or dexamphetamine, but rather less potent, and is used in children who are hyperkinetic or epileptic, to increase alertness. Pemoline is less likely to produce dependence and is longer-acting, so that once-daily dosage is enough

(0.5–2.0 mg/kg, or usually 20–80 mg daily, for children of 6–15 years). Begin with 20 mg daily and increase by 20 mg weekly, until the best response is achieved.

It does not interact with MAOI drugs but otherwise is like dexamphetamine, but less toxic.

It is not controlled under the Misuse of Drugs Act.

Preparations

Tablets: 20 mg.

Fenfluramine

Fenfluramine (Ponderax Pacaps) is chiefly used for suppression of appetite in the obese (see p. 127).

The dose by sustained-release capsule is 60 mg daily, raised to 120 mg and then 180 mg at two-week intervals, if necessary. Treatment must stop at eight weeks, with step-wise reduction every few days, to avoid risk of abuse or dependence.

Tiredness, sedation, diarrhoea, dizziness and headache are the most likely side-effects, and tolerance is possible. The drug can potentiate drugs used in the treatment of hypertension and also interacts with MAOIs with risk of excitement and hypertensive crisis. It is therefore best avoided when other medical treatments are necessary.

Preparations

Capsules (slow release): 60 mg.

24 Neuroleptics

These are drugs used primarily in the treatment of schizophrenia, and for mania, and are therefore sometimes called 'antipsychotics'. However, some may be used as hypnotics, or in small doses against anxiety and tension. They contrast clinically with the tricyclic antidepressants. Chemically they form several distinct groups. The phenothiazines and the thioxanthenes resemble the tricyclics in having a three-ring structure, but the central ring has six atoms instead of seven and one of them is sulphur: the type drugs are chlorpromazine and flupenthixol respectively. Then there are the butyrophenones (type: haloperidol) related to the analgesic pethidine, and the phenylbutyl piperidines (type: pimozide); and the dibenzamide sulpiride. Most recently dibenzoxapines have also been introduced.

Such a variety of active chemical structures implies differences in pharmacokinetic and metabolic activity. Although all appear to block dopamine receptors, and some are anticholinergic or have actions against other neurotransmitters, it is probable that they do not act all in the same ways on the central nervous system. In the clinic, therefore, if a member of one group fails to make sufficient impact on the patient's symptoms, a member of another group may do much better, and experimental changes of prescription are justified and worthwhile.

In the control of schizophrenia these drugs have to be taken regularly for months and years. Regular tablet-taking several times a day for such long periods is difficult and, therefore, depot preparations of the drugs are used, providing smooth cover from one intramuscular injection every two or four weeks. When converting from oral daily to intramuscular treatment the following very *rough* dosage guide may be useful:

fluphenazine to fluphenazine decanoate (Modecate) each 10 mg daily to 25 mg i.m. two-weekly
haloperidol to haloperidol decanoate (Haldol) each 30 mg daily to 100 mg i.m. four-weekly
flupenthixol to flupenthixol decanoate (Depixol) each 10 mg daily to 50 mg i.m. two-weekly
zuclopenthixol to zuclopenthixol decanoate (Clopixol) each 10 mg daily to 100 mg i.m. two-weekly.

These are the most used, but the phenothiazine/pipothiazine palmitate (Piportil) and the butylpiperidine fluspirilene (Redeptin) are also available for injection, while oral pimozide need not be taken every day in maintenance treatment. See the entries on individual drugs.

According to Tantam & McGrath (1989), 100 mg chlorpromazine or thioridazine roughly equal 2 mg fluphenazine, 3 mg flupenthixol or 2.5 mg haloperidol; or 5 mg trifluoperazine, 8 mg perphenazine, or 15 mg prochlorperazine.

Phenothiazines

This bewilderingly large group of drugs, of which chlorpromazine was the first to be used in psychiatry, all have molecular structures on the same ground plan (Fig. 4) and broadly similar effects, including blocking of dopamine receptors. The modifications to the molecule which vary the

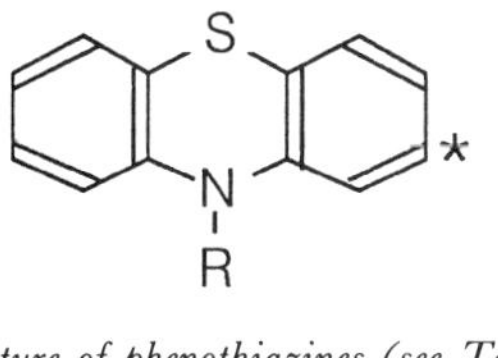

S
N
R
*

Fig. 4. The basic structure of phenothiazines (see Table 2)

TABLE 2

Variations on the phenothiazine ground plan
(the doses in milligrams are roughly equipotent for 1 mg fluphenazine)

Atom or atoms at R (side-chain)	*Atom or atoms at asterisk in Fig. 4*			
	–H	*–Cl*	*$-CF_3$*	*$-SCH_3$*
$-CH_2CH_2CH_2N(CH_3)_2$	Promazine	Chlorpromazine (100 mg)	Triflupromazine (40 mg)	
$-CH_2CH(CH_3)N(CH_3)_2$	Promethazine (300 mg)			
$-CH_2CH_2CH_2N\langle\,\rangle NCH_3$ 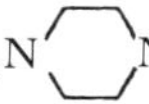		Prochlorperazine (30 mg)	Trifluoperazine (10 mg)	
$-CH_2CH_2CH_2N\langle\,\rangle NCH_2CH_2OH$ 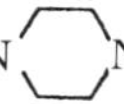		Perphenazine (10 mg)	Fluphenazine (1 mg)	
$-CH_2CH_2-\langle\,\rangle N-CH_3$ 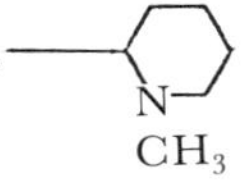				Thioridazine (100 mg)

clinical effects are in the atoms attached at the asterisk and the side-chain 'R' in Fig. 4. The liability to induce sleep, for instance, or Parkinsonism, is altered by changing 'R'. Particular 'R's also produce the depot phenothiazines. Alterations at the asterisk chiefly increase the potency of a given weight of drug without altering the antimanic or antischizophrenic actions. Table 2 will help an understanding of the inter-relations of some commonly used phenothiazines. The numbers indicate, very roughly, the number of milligrams of each substance having about the same clinical effect (but see p. 163). Drugs with the first type of side-chain in Table 2 (e.g. promethazine and chlorpromazine) have strong hypnotic properties; those with the second type of side-chain have no hypnotic action, but are more likely to produce Parkinsonism. The risk of Parkinsonism is greater still with the third type, which also has the most anti-emetic action, but liability to Parkinsonism is almost absent in the fourth type (thioridazine), perhaps because of its anticholinergic potency.

Long-acting fluphenazine decanoate (Modecate) is made by esterifying the 'R' side-chain terminal (OH) with a long-chain fatty acid (decanoic acid), which delays inactivation of the drug. A single intramuscular dose may be effective for up to four weeks.

All the drugs are rapidly metabolised in the liver by oxidation of the sulphur atom in the central ring, by hydroxylation of the side rings and by changes in the side-chains. Most of these metabolites are clinically inactive. Sulphoxides and hydroxy derivatives are excreted to some extent in urine but predominantly through the liver into the gut and then into the faeces. Note that the microbial flora of the gut is capable of reducing inactive sulphoxide back to active drug, which can then be reabsorbed and circulate again (so the health of the gut can modify the duration of phenothiazine action). Drug metabolites appear to be excreted for some months after drug-taking has stopped.

There is much variation from patient to patient in the speed of metabolism of the same drug. In some, metabolism begins in the gut wall even before absorption into the body. Metabolism is speeded up after two to three weeks of continued use; many drugs are then more rapidly destroyed and the same dose is, therefore, perhaps less effective. Remember that for pharmacokinetic reasons injected drug is three times more effective than oral, and syrup is more effective than tablet.

The elderly are much more sensitive to phenothiazines, therefore use smaller doses and less potent drugs. Normal and neurotic adults become drowsy on small doses that would not affect a schizophrenic or manic patient. An allergic reaction, for instance eczema, dermatitis, jaundice or other unusual physical response to one phenothiazine may indicate the need to try another. Brain-damaged patients may be unusually sensitive to phenothiazines. The tendency to have fits may be slightly increased in epilepsy, but the drugs are valuable for controlling the special irritability and aggression which sometimes occur in epilepsy.

For control of psychotic illnesses it is best not to be timid or tentative but to start with quite big doses – 100 mg chlorpromazine or 10 mg trifluoperazine, each thrice daily – and soon adjust the dose as required. The occasional patient finds the acute dose too big and rather quickly develops a dystonic reaction, which may be misjudged as hysterical – writhing body movements, arching of the back, torticollis, protruding lolling tongue. This can be treated by adjusting the dose and with anti-Parkinsonian drugs (see p. 183).

Where one phenothiazine in full dosage as syrup or by injection has not been successful, another is unlikely to do much better. It is preferable to change to a butyrophenone or a thioxanthene. These drugs are chemically quite distinct from the phenothiazines, although similar in effect. All these drugs take time, even several weeks of continuous administration, to abolish schizophrenic symptoms but are quick to control mania.

With high doses of neuroleptics continued for some time, especially in the elderly, a state of muscular rigidity with fever, sweating, a raised serum creatinine phosphokinase, and fluctuating pulse rate and blood pressure, is sometimes (but rarely) encountered. If concurrent acute physical illness can be excluded with certainty, this may be an example of the controversial 'neuroleptic malignant syndrome' (pp. 38, 39). If the neuroleptics are stopped, and the patient treated with attention to fluid balance and pyrexia, the condition usually remits in five to ten days (possibly longer with depot drugs). Some advocate 5–15 mg bromocriptine daily to relieve the muscular rigidity. Some consider the prognosis of this syndrome to be poor but the sometimes unrecognised complications of pulmonary infection or toxic interaction of drugs have produced confusion among observers, and uncertainty.

Chlorpromazine

Chlorpromazine (Largactil) may be used for:

(a) severe disturbance, whatever the cause
(b) control and maintenance therapy of schizophrenia
(c) insomnia
(d) nausea, vomiting
(e) anorexia nervosa, as an appetite stimulant
(f) tension and anxiety.

For acutely disturbed states chlorpromazine is the classic drug of choice (equal with haloperidol), having a prolonged quietening effect without impairment of consciousness. Chlorpromazine is therefore used to control manic states, acutely disturbed schizophrenics, delirium and confusional states, to cover drug withdrawal in the drug dependent, and to prevent outbursts in the aggressive epileptic. Large doses are tolerated and indeed required, since to gain control quickly is important. Chlorpromazine syrup (100 mg) repeated every four to six hours for three to six doses usually achieves control; initially, in the most severe, a deep intramuscular injection of 100 mg repeated as necessary is recommended, converting (by overlapping) to an oral dose as soon as co-operation is achieved. Tranquillising effects should be evident within 6–24 hours and doses of 300–800 mg a day continued. Once the abnormal behaviour is controlled, start reducing the dose.

Acute disturbance apart, chlorpromazine is invaluable for the treatment of schizophrenia, especially paranoid and catatonic types. The antipsychotic effect begins after three to six days and delusions lessen, auditory hallucinations diminish or cease and thought disorder is less marked. Start with 150 mg oral chlorpromazine daily, which may need to be raised in 150 mg daily steps, at intervals, up to 900 mg for control. Increasing the dose too quickly in the initial stages may induce dystonic reaction; a high dose at two to three weeks may induce Parkinsonism; very long continued treatment causes other unwanted effects.

A dose of 50–100 mg at night produces an early hypnotic effect. Small doses (25–50 mg three times daily) reduce nausea and vomiting, and similar doses or higher are used in anorexia nervosa to stimulate appetite and weight gain. Where minor tranquillisers might be used, 10–25 mg three times daily suppresses tension and anxiety in neurotic states; higher doses can lessen obsession.

Early side-effects

(a) Common: sedation, hypotension (dizziness), dry or nasty mouth, indigestion, blurred vision, all usually improving as soon as tolerance spontaneously develops.

(b) Rare: dystonia – sudden appearance of torticollis, arching of back, tongue protrusion, writhing, abnormal movements or oculogyric crisis, all suggestive of hysterical reaction or onset of acute neurological damage. Treat by temporary reduction in chlorpromazine dosage, since the condition is reversible, and by giving of parenteral anti-Parkinsonian drugs. Diazepam can be given as well to control anxiety. Relief begins in about 10 minutes.

Medium-term side-effects

(a) Mild skin rash at 21 days is trivial, and quickly fades.

(b) Tiredness, weakness, internal restlessness (akathisia or 'jitters'), insomnia at night though drowsy by day, and Parkinsonism developing – stiffness of arms and legs, of cramps, loss of facial mobility and expression, sometimes salivation. These are not spontaneously resolving. Treat with anti-Parkinsonian drugs or by reduction of phenothiazine dose.

(c) Weight gain, by degrees, of 6 kg or more to a plateau. Reverses slowly when phenothiazine is stopped; dieting is recommended.

(d) Galactorrhoea can be distressing but has to be tolerated. Sometimes amenorrhoea occurs.

(e) Some patients on chlorpromazine are liable to easy sunburn in summer. Avoid direct exposure (use shady hats and gloves) and use Uvistat, or other ultraviolet-blocking skin cream. Consider changing to thioridazine, which does not cause photosensitivity.

(f) Pigmentation of exposed skin is more of a risk for women because they have more exposed skin in the summer.

(g) Fingers are more liable to freezing and frostbite in very cold weather, and patients should wear warm gloves when outside.

(h) Occasional epileptic fits can be treated with anticonvulsants.

(i) Jaundice: there is possibly an increased risk of contracting infective hepatitis, also obstructive (cholestatic) jaundice. Stop chlorpromazine, treat liver complaint, later resume with a different phenothiazine.

(j) Agranulocytosis can occur, though rarely, and lead to death.

Late side-effects: tardive dyskinesia

After two years or more of continuous drug treatment, especially on the higher doses and in the elderly, or where there is brain damage (neurological disease, leucotomy, dementia), rhythmic spontaneous movements appear, especially around the mouth and in the tongue. Stopping the drug may allow the abnormal movements to disappear. Continuing the drug is not necessarily associated with a worsening of the condition; prognosis is a very individual matter, not understood. Tetrabenazine, a chemical relative of reserpine, may be worth a trial to control tardive dyskinesia.

Contraindications and interactions

Chlorpromazine is compatible with all drugs and with electroconvulsive therapy (ECT).

Chlorpromazine stimulates liver drug metabolism after about two weeks of use, thereby arranging its own quicker destruction, and the quicker destruction of a number of other drugs, which will then have to be given in higher dosage. The increased rate of metabolism declines in about two weeks on stopping phenothiazines.

Chlorpromazine blocks the liver metabolism of some drugs, such as morphine, pethidine, and tricyclic antidepressants, which may then have more prolonged actions without change of dose.

Chlorpromazine is contraindicated where the patient is already semicomatose from barbiturates or alcohol, or is known to suffer from liver disease such as cirrhosis, or immediately following an attack of hepatitis. Where there is a history of a previous allergic response to chlorpromazine, it will be better to try a different phenothiazine, for example trifluoperazine.

Large doses may diminish symptoms of acute abdominal conditions and of fevers, making physical diagnosis harder.

Preparations

Tablets: 10 mg, 25 mg, 50 mg, 100 mg
Syrup: 25 mg/5 ml
Forte suspension: 100 mg/5 ml
Intramuscular injection: 25 mg/ml in 1 ml and 2 ml ampoules
Suppositories: 100 mg

Thioridazine

Thioridazine (Melleril) is particularly useful in calming agitation and restlessness but otherwise is used for the same purposes and in the same doses as chlorpromazine, although there is no injectable form.

Of all phenothiazines, thioridazine is the least likely to produce extrapyramidal signs, probably because of its pronounced anticholinergic properties (compare anti-Parkinsonian drugs). Dizziness and muzziness resulting from hypotension, especially postural hypotension, may occur, particularly at the start of treatment. Use smaller doses, raise the dose more gradually, or change to another phenothiazine. Doses above 600 mg a day, particularly for long periods, should be avoided. Such a dose carries the risk of pigmentary retinopathy and blindness.

Preparations

Tablets: 10 mg, 25 mg, 50 mg, 100 mg
Syrup: 25 mg/5 ml
Suspension: 25 mg/5 ml and 100 mg/5 ml.

Promazine

Promazine (Sparine) is much less potent than chlorpromazine; it is used as a hypnotic or sedative for the elderly where drug-induced confusional states are a risk. Beware of producing over-sedation, urinary and faecal incontinence, or disorientation.

Orally give 25–100 mg once, or up to four times daily; intramuscularly give 50 mg, repeatable after six hours.

Preparations

Suspension: 50 mg/5 ml
Injection: 50 mg/ml in 1 ml and 2 ml ampoules.

Trifluoperazine

Trifluoperazine (Stelazine) is about ten times more potent, weight for weight, than chlorpromazine, is not a hypnotic, does not cause weight gain, but is strong in inducing Parkinsonism. Its indications are as for chlorpromazine.

Give 5–15 mg thrice daily by mouth; 1–5 mg once or more daily for symptomatic anxiety. Do not prescribe anti-Parkinsonian drugs routinely, but be ready to give them at once if they are needed. Review the question of need after two, four and eight weeks of continuous treatment, since the need may disappear as the psychosis settles, or if the phenothiazine dose is reduced for maintenance treatment.

Preparations

Tablets: 1 mg, 5 mg
Slow-release capsules: 2 mg, 10 mg, 15 mg
Syrup: 1 mg/5 ml
Concentrate: 10 mg/ml
Injection: 1 mg/ml, in 1 ml ampoules.

Perphenazine

The use and side-effects of perphenazine (Fentazin) are as for chlorpromazine, but it is less sedative and more prone to Parkinsonism.

Give 4–8 mg thrice daily as tablets, or 10 mg by intramuscular injection, and then repeating 5 mg six-hourly.

For anxiety, give 2 mg twice or thrice daily, and upwards. It has also been successfully used for intractable hiccough.

Preparations

Tablets: 2 mg, 4 mg.

Pericyazine

Pericyazine (Neulactil) is used for treating psychoses and behavioural disturbance, in doses of 15–30 mg by mouth for psychoses but up to 75 mg daily for severe behavioural disturbance due to psychoses or mental handicap.

Side-effects are as for chlorpromazine but pericyazine is more sedative.

Preparations

Tablets: 2.5 mg, 10 mg, 25 mg
Syrup: 10 mg/5 ml.

Related phenothiazines

Methotrimeprazine (Nozinan) –
tablets: 25 mg (maximum daily dose 200 mg)
Prochlorperazine (Stemetil) –
tablets: 5 mg, 25 mg (maximum daily dose 100 mg)
syrup: 5 mg/5 ml
granules: 5 mg in sachet.

Depot preparations: fluphenazine esters

Fluphenazine as the hydrochloride and sold as Moditen or Prolixin is the most potent phenothiazine weight for weight, and may be used orally whenever a phenothiazine seems suitable treatment. Modecate and Moditen enanthate are fluphenazine esterified in the side-chain with long-chain fatty acids (decanoic acid, oenanthoic acid) and dissolved in sesame oil for injection. A single dose will give therapeutic benefit for one to four weeks. The injected drug is transferred to fatty storage sites, then slowly released and metabolised, which accounts for long-lasting effects. The injection is therefore eminently suitable for long-term treatment of chronic schizophrenia, particularly in out-patients, who may not be able, or willing, particularly if they feel well, to take tablets regularly for very long periods, or for patients suspicious of tablets. It is also useful in preventing frequent recurrent attacks of mania or hypomania.

Fluphenazine need only be taken orally once a day in a dose of 1–10 mg. At least 5 mg is required to treat a psychosis. 'Modecate' (25 mg/1 ml) is given by deep intramuscular injection into the gluteal muscle once every two, three or four weeks at the start. With the elderly or the small patient, a test dose of 0.5 ml (12.5 mg) may be preferred, but it is not necessary as a routine. Muscular stiffness and cramps, tremor and restlessness may appear in the two days after injection, and reach a peak of severity at about five days and then die away. Such side-effects may require anti-Parkinsonian drugs or diazepam, or both, but only give them when they are clearly needed and not automatically. Side-effects can sometimes be avoided by halving the dose and giving the injection twice as often. Minor degrees of side-effects, especially drowsiness or flatness, and restlessness, are not uncommon and it may take some months for them to resolve.

The dose of Modecate which suppresses psychotic symptoms may be much more than 25 mg – perhaps even up to 175 mg. It can be difficult to decide how often to repeat the injection. Sometimes, in an otherwise well controlled patient, symptoms begin to reappear towards the end of the third week after the injection, which is a sign to shorten the interval between injections, or to increase the dose a little. The aim is to find the optimal interval and the smallest dose that will achieve control. Intervals longer than one month tend to be too long. Decide on a fixed interval, such as every two weeks, and then reduce the size of dose every month or six weeks (every second or third injection) gradually, watching for the reappearance of the original psychotic symptoms. Most will do well on 25 mg (1 ml) fortnightly; some manage on even less – 5 mg or 10 mg. Patients feel better on lower doses, have less Parkinsonism, and less risk of tardive dyskinesia. The patient should therefore be regularly and not too infrequently supervised by a therapist for observation of changes in mental state and side-effects. It is best done by an experienced doctor.

Preparations

Tablets: 1 mg, 2.5 mg, 5 mg

Fluphenazine decanoate (Modecate)
  injection (25 mg/ml): 0.5 ml, 1.0 ml, 2.0 ml ampoules
  ready-filled disposable 1.0 ml and 2.0 ml syringes
Fluphenazine decanoate (Modecate concentrate)
  injection (100 mg/ml): 0.5 ml, 1.0 ml ampoules
Fluphenazine enanthate (Moditen)
  injection (25 mg/ml): 1.0 ml ampoule.

Thioxanthenes

Thioxanthenes resemble phenothiazines closely, but have a carbon atom in place of the nitrogen atom of the middle ring to which the side-chain is attached. The side-chain is usually linked to this carbon by a double bond, which makes the molecule look a little like a tricyclic antidepressant with a sulphur atom (but a six-atom, not a seven-atom, central ring). The thioxanthene analogue of chlorpromazine is chlorprothixene (Taractan); flupenthixol is the analogue of fluphenazine, while zuclopenthixol has a chlorine atom, as does chlorprothixene, but a side-chain like flupenthixol.

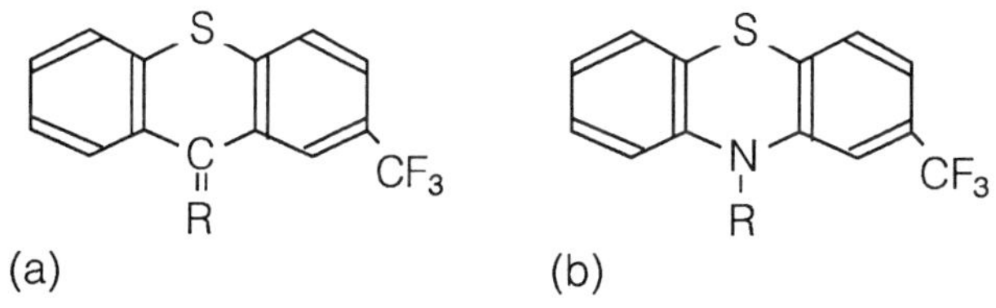

Fig. 5. Thioxanthene and phenothiazine compared: (a) flupenthixol, (b) fluphenazine

Flupenthixol

By deep intramuscular injection, flupenthixol is effective against schizophrenic symptoms (20–100 mg every 2–4 weeks), comparable with Modecate but less sedative. Begin with a test intramuscular dose of 20 mg and increase dose every 7–14 days. Rarely, doses can go up to 1600 mg fortnightly. The long-acting injection may also be tried to control mania when other treatments have failed (40–80 mg weekly). If successful it may be continued, to prevent relapse. Like other major tranquillisers, oral flupenthixol (Fluanxol) can be given in small doses (0.5–1.5 mg morning and midday) for anxiety and the higher-dose tablet (Depixol) be used to suppress a psychosis (3–9 mg twice daily).

Extrapyramidal effects are less common than with phenothiazines. A few patients become overactive.

Preparations

Flupenthixol –
  tablets: Fluanxol 0.5 mg, 1 mg
    Depixol 3 mg
Flupenthixol decanoate (Depixol)
  ampoules (clear): 20 mg in 1 ml, 40 mg in 2 ml
Flupenthixol decanoate (Depixol conc.)
  ampoules (amber): 100 mg in 1 ml.

Zuclopenthixol

Zuclopenthixol (Clopixol) is more sedative than flupenthixol and has about one-fifth the potency, allowing a finer adjustment to the best dose. For maintenance in schizophrenia, start with 100 mg deep intramuscular gluteal injection and increase to 200–500 mg over four weeks. For aggressive behaviour, give 20–50 mg orally daily, but initially higher doses, of up to 150 mg daily, may be required.

Preparations

Zuclopenthixol di HCl (oral)
  tablets: 2 mg, 10 mg, 25 mg
Zuclopenthixol decanoate (Clopixol)
  injection (200 mg/ml): 1.0 ml ampoule, 10 ml vial
  injection (500 mg/ml): 1.0 ml ampoule with needle.

Butyrophenones and piperidines

These drugs, related chemically to the analgesic pethidine, are mostly used in psychiatry for the control of schizophrenia, mania and acute brain syndrome, especially when aggression and excitement are present. They block dopamine receptors. Although chemically quite distinct from phenothiazines, their effects are very similar, but some individual patients may do better with one type of drug than with the other. Some are long-acting, presumably because they are slowly metabolised and excreted. Haloperidol is the type drug (Fig. 6). Chemical modifications result in pimozide and fluspirilene, which need not be taken every day.

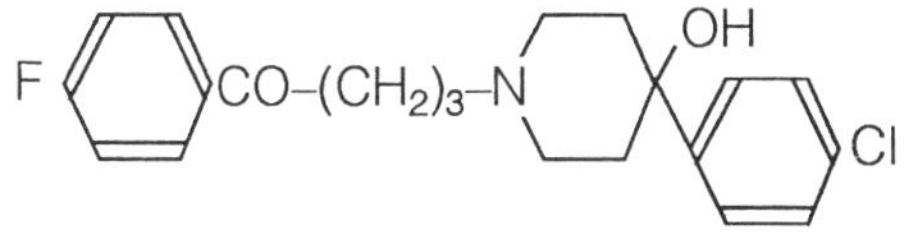

Fig. 6. The structure of haloperidol

Haloperidol

Haloperidol (Serenace, Haldol, Dozic, Fortunan) may be used for:

(a) severe excitement and overactivity
(b) continued treatment of mania and schizophrenia
(c) chronic anxiety states
(d) Gilles de la Tourette's syndrome.

For the acutely excited and overactive patient, begin with 5–10 mg intramuscularly, repeated two-hourly up to 60 mg total over 12 hours if necessary. This dosage controls most states, and when it does the dose can be reduced to 5–10 mg thrice daily orally and then further reduced in a few days depending on the response. Because of side-effects, 10 mg oral procyclidine thrice daily may need to be given. If intravenous haloperidol is given, then 10 mg intravenous procyclidine may be given at the same time but in a separate syringe. These high doses of haloperidol are required in manic, drug-induced, and schizophrenic excitements, but lower doses may be quite adequate for acute brain syndromes.

In continued treatment for mania and schizophrenia, 3–5 mg thrice daily is usually adequate, but a frequent check for psychotic symptoms and side-effects should guide. For schizophrenics larger doses may be needed and may be well tolerated. Claims are made that doses up to 80 mg a day are effective in resistant cases, but this is not yet accepted practice. More often the drug is now used in depot form for maintenance therapy.

For chronic anxiety states give 0.5 mg twice daily, but benzodiazepines are preferable in the short term since they are equally effective and have less severe side-effects. Children with Gilles de la Tourette's syndrome should be maintained on the lower effective dose, which is likely to be around 0.1 mg/kg a day. Pimozide (see below) is a good alternative (0.05–0.20 mg/kg).

Side-effects

Extrapyramidal effects are common, more so than with chlorpromazine, and can occur at any stage of giving the drug. Stiffness, rigidity or extreme restlessness are the most frequent. The elderly and those with basal ganglia disease are especially prone to extrapyramidal effects.

Side-effects can occur with remarkable suddenness even after a single small dose, though are more likely with larger doses. They may appear as excitement lessens. Side-effects may persist for three months or longer after stopping haloperidol (see pp. 53, 54). Intravenous procyclidine (10 mg) relieves acute symptoms. Oral anti-Parkinsonian drugs are given only when side-effects appear. Test at intervals, by their gradual withdrawal, whether they continue to be needed during long-term treatment.

Preparations

Tablets: 1.5 mg, 5 mg, 10 mg, 20 mg
Capsules: 0.5 mg
Liquid: 2 mg/ml, 10 mg/ml
Injection: 5 mg/1 ml; 10 mg/1 ml; and 20 mg/2 ml.

Haloperidol decanoate in oil –
ampoules: 50 mg/1 ml; 100 mg/1 ml.

Related drugs

Trifluperidol ('Triperidol') –
tablets: 0.5 mg, 1 mg (maximum daily dose 8 mg)
Benperidol ('Anquil') –
tablets: 0.25 mg (maximum daily dose 1.5 mg)
Droperidol ('Droleptan') –
tablets: 10 mg
liquid: 1 mg/ml
injection: 5 mg/ml in 2 ml ampoule
Use as for haloperidol and in similar dosage.

Pimozide

Pimozide (Orap) may be used for:

(a) schizophrenia
(b) mania
(c) chronic anxiety
(d) Gilles de la Tourette's syndrome
(e) monosymptomatic hypochondriasis.

For acute psychosis it is given once daily in a starting dose of 10 mg, which can be increased by weekly steps of 2 mg or 4 mg to 20 mg. For other indications start with 2 mg and increase gradually in 2 mg steps to a maximum of 16 mg. Its advantages are: (a) that it is fairly free of all side-effects, so that patients find it agreeable; Parkinsonism is uncommon, and mild, but there may be some drowsiness and possibly hypotension; and (b) it has a long elimination half-life, which means its plasma concentration changes rather slowly, and even omitting a day's dose will not alter the level much. However, it is contraindicated if there is any history of cardiac arrhythmia or a prolonged QT in the electrocardiogram (ECG). An ECG should be done before starting treatment. Avoid other neuroleptics, cardioactive drugs, or hepatic/renal disease and hypokalaemia.

For children with Gilles de la Tourette's syndrome give 0.05–0.20 mg/kg per day. For hypochondriasis and anxiety try small doses (2 mg daily).

Preparations

Tablets: 2 mg, 4 mg, 10 mg.

Fluspirilene

Fluspirilene (Redeptin) is an injectable piperidine for psychosis. Begin with 2 mg per week, rising by 2 mg weekly to a maximum if needed of 20 mg.

Preparations

Solution: 2 mg/ml in 1 ml, 2 ml ampoules, 6 ml vial.

Unclassified neuroleptics

Sulpiride

Sulpiride (Dolmatil, Sulpitil) was introduced about ten years ago; this chemically totally distinct drug (Fig. 7) is said to have antidepressant activity in its lower doses (below 200 mg daily) and antischizophrenic activity at higher levels, when it is also sedative.

It is not metabolised to any extent but excreted unchanged in the urine. Parkinsonism, if present, is mild, anticholinergic

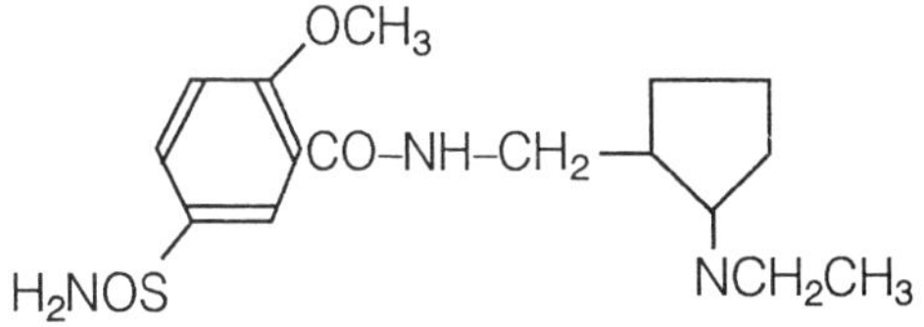

Fig. 7. The structure of sulpiride

side-effects minimal, and reports of tardive dyskinesia are so far rare. Poisoning by overdose can result in restlessness and clouding of consciousness, leading to coma and low blood pressure, but there have been no deaths and recovery is quick.

For positive schizophrenic symptoms, start with 400 mg twice daily rising quickly to a maximum of 1200 mg twice daily. For negative symptoms try reducing the dose from 400 mg towards 200 mg. In general, do not change dose more often than once per week.

Preparations

Tablets: 200 mg.

Oxypertine

Oxypertine (Integrin) is chiefly used for psychosis. Start with 80 mg daily, rising to a maximum of 300 mg.

Preparations

Capsules: 10 mg
Tablets: 40 mg.

Clozapine

Clozapine (Clozaril), a dibenzodiazepine neuroleptic, is claimed to be effective in schizophrenia resistant to treatment by other neuroleptics and to have a different neurotransmitter-blocking pattern, notably a weaker antidopaminergic action and less strongly Parkinsonian. It is said to combine well with haloperidol, which has some complementary actions.

Unfortunately it is prone to cause agranulocytosis, which can be fatal. Any patient put on clozapine must be registered with the "Clozaril Patient Monitoring Service" (Sandoz, tel. 0276-692255), and have weekly leucocyte counts thereafter, to reduce the risks. Tachycardia may be pronounced.

Dosage is 25 mg daily, increasing each day by 25 mg to a maximum of 200–450 mg daily (in divided doses); full contraindications and side-effects should be known before starting. Neutropenia is a sign to stop.

Preparations

Tablets: 25 mg, 100 mg.

Loxapine

Loxapine (Loxapac) is another dibenzoxazepine neuroleptic, with risks of dystonia, Parkinsonism, epileptic fits, hypotension, and loss of alertness. The recommended dose is 10 mg twice daily, rising over ten days to a daily total of 80–100 mg.

Preparations

Capsules: 10 mg, 25 mg, 50 mg.

Reference

TANTAM, D. & MCGRATH, G. (1989) Prolonged use of neuroleptics in schizophrenia: a review for the practitioner. *International Clinical Psychopharmacology*, **4**, 167–194.

25 Anti-Parkinsonian drugs

Extrapyramidal symptoms encountered in psychiatric practice are nearly all drug-induced (see under "Extrapyramidal reactions", p. 82). Only a small number result from primary basal ganglia disease. Phenothiazines with a piperazine side-chain (R in Table 2, p. 164, e.g. trifluoperazine) and the butyrophenones are the two groups of antipsychotic drugs that most commonly cause Parkinsonism and other extrapyramidal syndromes. On occasion, tricyclic antidepressants in high dose may also be responsible; with lower doses, adding lithium will also provoke such reactions.

Parkinson's disease itself was first successfully treated with the atropine group of drugs, which block cholinergic activity. Subsequently atropine-like synthetic drugs, also antihistaminic in action, were developed, and then drugs which increased the effectiveness of natural basal ganglia dopamine, such as L-dopa and amantadine. Neither of these latter drugs is useful in drug-induced Parkinsonism, but they are relevant to psychiatric practice because of their side-effects or their occasional use for primary Parkinsonism in psychiatric patients. Fifteen per cent of patients taking L-dopa develop significant psychiatric symptoms and may present to the psychiatrist with a toxic confusional state (acute brain syndrome), depression, hypomania, or paranoid state; L-dopa has then to be reduced or stopped. Amantadine is less of a problem, but in a few patients, especially those who have had a previous psychiatric illness, psychotic states with confusion and hallucinations occur.

The synthetic anticholinergic drugs benzhexol, benztropine and procyclidine and antihistaminics like orphenadrine can control or modify drug-induced extrapyramidal disorders so that antipsychotic medication may be maintained. Anti-Parkinsonian drugs should not be prescribed routinely to patients on antipsychotic drugs, but only when substantial and persistent side-effects appear. The psychotropic action of phenothiazines may be modified and the early stages of tardive dyskinesia masked by anti-Parkinsonian drugs. If extrapyramidal symptoms do appear, consider reducing the level of antipsychotic drug before prescribing anti-Parkinsonian drugs.

The synthetic anticholinergic drugs used in large doses, especially in the elderly, can produce an acute brain syndrome. Their anticholinergic activity can interfere with the treatment of glaucoma, and provoke acute retention of urine in men with prostatic hypertrophy. Side-effects may appear before the optimal dose for controlling Parkinsonian symptoms is achieved. Benzhexol is discussed in some detail as the type drug and others described briefly.

Benzhexol

Benzhexol (Artane, Bentex, Broflex) is occasionally used in early stages of idiopathic Parkinsonism but largely for drug-induced extrapyramidal symptoms. Benzhexol relieves drug-induced akinesia, rigidity, dystonic reactions, and tremor to less extent. The usual effective dose lies between 5 mg and 15 mg daily. Start with a low dose (1 mg daily) and increase slowly, giving the drug two or three times a day, until control of symptoms is achieved or new side-effects become more of a problem to the patient than the extrapyramidal symptoms. Several days should be allowed to elapse between each increase of the dose to allow tolerance to develop. The patient may eventually tolerate several times the initial dose.

Side-effects include drowsiness and nausea, resulting from the central action of the drug, and blurred vision, dry mouth, constipation and urinary difficulties, the result of peripheral action of the drug, may limit the use of high doses. On the other hand, some patients experience a pleasurable 'buzz' which leads them on to higher doses and addiction.

The central action of high doses may also cause an acute brain syndrome similar to atropine intoxication, with delirium, hallucinations and confusion. The elderly and those with cerebral impairment are more at risk of such a side-effect, and so try to keep to a low dose. The anticholinergic effect at the periphery may precipitate an attack of acute glaucoma, interfere with the treatment of chronic glaucoma, and cause urinary retention in men with prostatic hypertrophy.

On the whole, side-effects diminish as tolerance to the drug develops. If they do not diminish, the dose should be reduced or an alternative drug tried.

Do not stop treatment abruptly, as this may precipitate acute side-effects (akinesia, rigidity, salivation, urinary retention).

Preparations

Tablets: 2 mg, 5 mg
Syrup: 5 mg/5 ml.

Benztropine

Benztropine (Cogentin) is used similarly for drug-induced extrapyramidal symptoms. The drug is cumulative, so it is better to start with a low dose (0.5 mg) once daily for the first few days and slowly increase the dose to 6 mg daily if necessary. Some patients do better on divided doses, some on a single daily dose.

Acute dystonic reactions are relieved by 2 mg given parenterally, but this may need to be repeated.

Preparations

Tablets: 2 mg
Injection: 2 mg/2 ml ampoule.

Procyclidine

Procyclidine (Arpicolin, Kemadrin) is widely used in psychiatric practice. The dose for Parkinsonian symptoms is 10–30 mg daily in divided doses depending on the response. Some patients experience a 'buzz' with the drug and become addicted, taking large amounts.

Procyclidine is the drug of choice for acute dystonic reactions, given parenterally, in a dose of 10–20 mg intramuscularly or 5–10 mg intravenously.

Preparations

Tablets: 5 mg
Syrup: 2.5 mg/5 ml, 5 mg/5 ml
Injection: 10 mg/2 ml ampoule.

Orphenadrine

Start orphenadrine (Biorphen, Disipal) at 100 mg per day, increasing to 300 mg in divided doses depending on response. It is generally well tolerated by patients.

Preparations

Tablets: 50 mg
Syrup: 25 mg/5 ml

Biperiden

Biperiden (Akineton) is similar to orphenadrine. Start with 2 mg daily doses and increase up to 12 mg daily.

Preparations

Tablets: 2 mg
Injection: 5 mg/ml.

Tetrabenazine

Tetrabenazine (Nitoman) is used for the control of abnormal movement disorders such as Huntington's chorea and tardive dyskinesia. Start with 25 mg thrice daily and increase by 25 mg a day every three days to a maximum of 200 mg total daily unless side-effects develop. If there is no improvement in symptoms after seven days of high-dose treatment, do not persist with the drug.

Do not give with a monoamine oxidase inhibitor because of the risk of an acute confusional state, and use cautiously in combination with L-dopa.

Drowsiness, indigestion, hypotension, and Parkinsonism when the drug is used in high dosage are all side-effects. If depression occurs, treat with a tricyclic.

Preparations

Tablets: 25 mg.

26 Benzodiazepines

Benzodiazepines are valuable hypnotics, anxiolytics or 'minor tranquillisers', and anticonvulsants. It is difficult to commit suicide with them in overdose when only they are taken, and they can safely be taken with other drugs without serious interactions. But rapid central nervous system tolerance results in dependence, and unpleasant symptoms on withdrawal. Abrupt withdrawal, after high dose or long use, can result in an acute brain syndrome, with disorientation and delirium, a paranoid psychosis and sometimes convulsions. Rapid withdrawal from low-dose treatment causes insomnia, anxiety, tremor, and sweating, symptoms similar to those for which the benzodiazepine may have been first prescribed, and these may last for days. In a few patients, such symptoms persist for months. Here a careful plan of slow and phased withdrawal, using diazepam, with concurrent group support and relaxation classes, is helpful.

Benzodiazepines are not harmless sedatives and hypnotics. They should be prescribed for a defined purpose within a plan of management. Prescribe for a finite period, for example two weeks, and then review their effects and only renew the prescription with justification. But at the same time it must be remembered that not every patient becomes dependent and, of those who do, not all take ever-increasing doses. Work with two or three from the large range of these drugs available and get to know a short-acting and a long-acting type.

Benzodiazepines are closely related compounds all with the same ring structure (Fig. 8) to which atoms or radicals like –H, –OH, $-CH_3$, –Cl can be attached at different points (Table 3). In metabolism, $-CH_3$ radicals can be removed

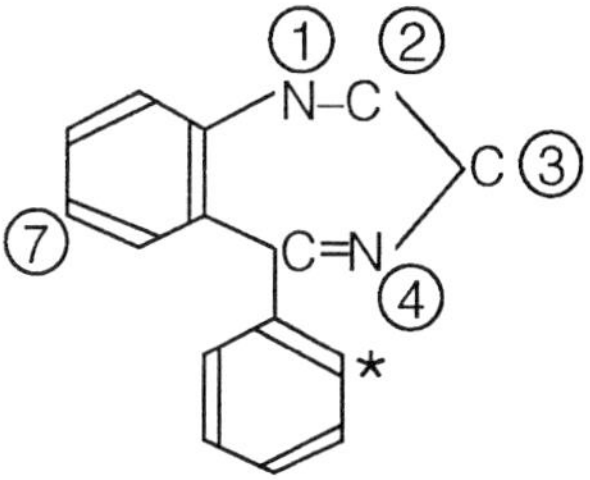

Fig. 8. The benzodiazepine structure

(demethylation) and the active drug is turned into another active substance – diazepam, medazepam, chlordiazepoxide and clorazepate all give rise to N-desmethyldiazepam, and this metabolite itself will have a long-term effect. Benzodiazepines differ among themselves chiefly in potency per mg, and in speed of inactivation and excretion. Temazepam for example is quickly converted to inactive glucuronide and excreted by the kidney and is therefore short-acting, and useful as a hypnotic. But diazepam is converted to

TABLE 3
Variations on the benzodiazepine ground plan

Drug	*Position (see Fig. 8)*					
	1	*2*	*3*	*4*	*7*	*
Chlordiazepoxide	–	$NH.CH_3$	H_2	O	Cl	–
Diazepam	CH_3	O	H_2	–	Cl	–
Medazepam	CH_3	H_2	H_2	–	Cl	–
Temazepam	CH_3	O	OH	–	Cl	–
Oxazepam	H	O	H.OH	–	Cl	–
Lorazepam	H	O	H.OH	–	Cl	Cl
Clonazepam	H	O	H_2	–	NO_2	Cl
Nitrazepam	H	O	H_2	–	NO_2	–
Flurazepam	$(CH_2)_2N(C_2H_5)_2$	O	H_2	–	Cl	F
Clorazepate	H	OH.OK	H.COOK	–	Cl	–
Triazolam	triazolo	–	–	Cl	Cl	–

Note that the first three structures give rise to oxazepam on oxidation and that lorazepam is chloro-oxazepam, as clonazepam is chloronitrazepam.

desmethyldiazepam, which is active and only slowly converted to inert substances. Physicochemical properties also play a part. Diazepam is absorbed from the gut more quickly than lorazepam, penetrates the brain more quickly, and comes out again more quickly, to spread into fat and muscles round the body. Lorazepam is slower to do these things; in consequence it acts for longer on the brain although it is more quickly eliminated from the body.

Difficulty in getting to sleep can be treated with a rapid-onset, short-acting benzodiazepine such as temazepam, or triazolam. The dose used is high relative to that for control of anxiety. After a good night's sedation the patient should wake fresh without hangover, drowsiness or dysphoria.

Large doses of short-acting benzodiazepines cause tolerance in 3–14 days. On stopping treatment two or three nights of insomnia will occur before natural sleep rhythm returns, and patients should be told this, otherwise they will ask for more drug. Be wary of using longer-acting benzodiazepines as the drugs accumulate and have effects the next day. Benzodiazepines are for short-term control of insomnia.

Episodes of acute anxiety can be prevented with a single dose of diazepam, which has both a rapid and a slow component of action. The patient must know the situations likely to provoke anxiety and should practise once or twice before they take place to get the dose and timing right. For example, 2 mg or 5 mg of diazepam by mouth taken one hour before a stressful interview might be helpful.

Persistent anxiety can be controlled or made tolerable with a regular low dose of a longer-acting benzodiazepine such as oxazepam or diazepam. Although lower doses produce tolerance less quickly than larger, dependence is still a risk and treatment should not be longer than four weeks. Since chronic anxiety usually fluctuates a good deal in severity, intermittent use of these drugs, which is preferable to daily use, is a practical course.

Benzodiazepines can cause impairment of mental ability, amnesia, decreased psychomotor skills and, in the elderly, ataxia. In some personalities they result in disinhibition and even aggression. Avoid prescribing for personalities prone to dependency. Alcohol and cimetidine both block benzodiazepine metabolism and interact centrally. Kidney and liver disease increase sensitivity. Benzodiazepines cause respiratory depression, particularly in the elderly, and those with emphysema and bronchitis are made worse by them.

Benzodiazepines still have a part to play in controlling human distress. Occasionally there will be circumstances where the evils of drug dependence are less than the disabling and painful symptoms of a psychiatric condition which cannot otherwise be ameliorated. A benzodiazepine may be better than alcohol, if that is the alternative for the patient. Diazepam is discussed in detail as the type drug; other benzodiazepines differ little from diazepam.

Diazepam

Diazepam (Alupram, Atensine, Tensium, Valium) may be used for:

(a) alleviation of anxiety
(b) treatment of insomnia
(c) relief of delirium tremens
(d) relief of LSD reactions
(e) abreaction
(f) control of status epilepticus.

A single oral dose of 5 mg or 10 mg, occasionally more, will dampen anxiety in half to one hour, or may be taken before an anxiety-provoking situation. This quick effect will wear off in about four hours. The drug is metabolised to a less potent but more persistent anxiolytic. Repeated doses of 2 mg or more can be given on a regular schedule twice or three times daily, or even more often, when the main benefit will come from the accumulation of the less potent metabolite, which is slow to build up and slow to disappear when treatment is stopped. Prescribe the smallest dose that will relieve symptoms. Avoid giving more than 30 mg per day and review the dosage weekly.

Diazepam can be used for insomnia, particularly when the problem is getting to sleep, but its metabolite may produce hangover effects next morning, especially when used on successive nights. Temazepam or triazolam are better. Assess critically whether patients taking regular daytime diazepam need separate night sedation or, likewise, whether patients taking regular night sedation need daytime sedation.

In acute stress, or to induce relaxation in a behavioural desensitisation programme, or in abreaction, 10 mg or even 20 mg can be given intramuscularly or intravenously.

For delirium tremens and for reactions to LSD, 10 mg parenterally is repeated until control is achieved, and then oral doses used to maintain control until the acute state has remitted.

Diazepam is the treatment of choice for status epilepticus (p. 107), by slow intravenous infusion or, in infants, by rectal infusion. Other benzodiazepines are not used in this way or in delirium tremens, but clonazepam can be a useful drug for epilepsy.

Side-effects and interactions

Tiredness or sleepiness may develop after some days, particularly on higher doses as can a morning hangover feeling. Ataxia and dizziness are less common. Pain in the legs has been noted in some elderly patients. Nausea and headache have been reported in others. In a very few patients aggressive behaviour appears. In some, anxiety may even be increased. Drug dependence may develop on higher doses and withdrawal symptoms appear a week or so after the drug is stopped. Sudden withdrawal may provoke fits.

Diazepam is less suitable for the elderly because of the greater risk of mental confusion and ataxia, or in the presence of cardiorespiratory disorders as respiration is depressed.

Preparations

Tablets: 2 mg, 5 mg, 10 mg
Capsules: 2 mg, 5 mg

Elixir: 2 mg/5 ml
Injection: 5 mg/ml
Rectal solution: 2 mg/ml, 4mg/ml
Suppositories: 10 mg.

Other anxiolytics

*Alprazolam (Xanax) –
  tablets: 0.25 mg, 0.5 mg (maximum daily dose 3 mg)
†Chlordiazepoxide (Librium, Tropium) –
  tablets: 5 mg, 10 mg, 25 mg (maximum daily dose 60 mg)
  capsules: 5 mg, 10 mg.
*Clobazam (Frisium) –
  capsules: 10 mg (maximum daily dose 30 mg)
*Clorazepate (Tranxene) –
  capsules: 7.5 mg, 15 mg (maximum daily dose 22.5 mg)
†Lorazepam (Ativan, Almazine) –
  tablets: 1 mg, 2.5 mg
  injection: 4 mg/ml (maximum daily dose 5 mg)
  withdrawal symptoms are common.
*Medazepam (Nobrium) –
  capsules: 5 mg, 10 mg (maximum daily dose 30 mg)
†Oxazepam (Oxanid) –
  tablets: 10 mg, 15 mg, 30 mg
  capsules: 30 mg (maximum daily dose 90 mg)
*Bromazepam (Lexotan) –
  tablets: 1.5 mg, 3 mg (maximum daily dose 18 mg)

Other hypnotics

Short-acting

Lormetazepam –
  tablets: 0.5, 1 mg (maximum daily dose 1 mg)

†Temazepam (Normison) –
tablets: 10 mg, 20 mg (maximum daily dose 30 mg)
capsules: 10 mg, 15 mg, 20 mg, 30 mg
elixir: 10 mg/5 ml.
†Triazolam (Halcion)
tablets: 0.125 mg, 0.250 mg (maximum daily dose 0.25 mg)

Longer-acting

†Nitrazepam (Mogadon, Remnos, Somnite, Unisomnia, Nitrados) –
tablets: 5 mg (maximum daily dose 10 mg)
capsules: 5 mg
mixture: 2.5 mg/5 ml
*Flunitrazepam (Rohypnol) –
tablets: 1 mg (maximum daily dose 1 mg)
*Flurazepam (Dalmane, Paxane) –
capsules: 15 mg, 30 mg (maximum daily dose 30 mg).

Note. The benzodiazepine brands marked with an asterisk are not available at NHS expense. Drugs marked with a dagger may only be prescribed under generic (not brand) names.

27 Barbiturates

Barbiturates are used in psychiatry for anaesthesia for electroconvulsive therapy, to control epilepsy, sometimes for abreaction, occasionally for narcosis, and only rarely for symptom control, because they carry serious risks of drug dependence and neuropsychiatric syndromes. The chronic use of barbiturates for the control of anxiety and sleeplessness is no longer justified. In our view barbiturates can be valuable as sedatives and hypnotics when used in cases where control is urgent and other tranquillisers have failed, but use should be limited to a few days. A small number of elderly people who have become dependent on regular doses of barbiturates remain an exception: it is best to let them continue.

Barbiturates are used both as the free acid (e.g. amylobarbitone) and as the sodium salt (e.g. sodium amylobarbitone). The acid is absorbed slowly because of its poor solubility. The salt has a faster action because of speedier absorption.

The different members of the barbiturate group vary principally in the speed with which they are metabolised by the liver and excreted in the urine; the more slowly metabolised barbiturates are more likely to cause hangovers and to accumulate. Accumulation can cause a chronic brain syndrome – drowsiness, disorientation, muddled thinking, slurred speech and ataxia. The elderly are especially liable because their bodies deal slowly with drugs. Barbiturates should be avoided in geriatric prescribing.

Barbiturates should not be given to children except for epilepsy (see p. 209) as they impair learning ability and cause disturbed behaviour. When tolerance develops, the same dose no longer relieves the symptoms. The doctor then has to consider whether to increase the dose to achieve control of symptoms, bearing in mind the risk of dependence, by stepwise increase of dose, or to stop barbiturates and use some other drug. In the dependent state the patient becomes irritable and moody whenever doses are not maintained. Cutting down the dose results in sleeplessness, agitation, complaints of tension, depression and even grand mal fits if the reduction is rapid. The drug must never be stopped abruptly, but the dose reduced slowly over about six weeks.

Amylobarbitone sodium

Amylobarbitone sodium (Sodium Amytal) is now used only rarely (and when major tranquillisers have failed) to control severe emotional and behavioural disturbance and for short periods of a few days. Start with 400 mg or 600 mg orally and then 200 mg four-hourly. More rapid control is gained by a single intramuscular or slow intravenous dose of 250 mg or more (up to 0.5 g i.m. or 1 g i.v.) the dose being judged by its almost immediate effect and repeated in a revised dose when the effect begins to wear off. Combined barbiturate and major tranquilliser can prove dramatically effective when the latter alone achieves little. For insomnia, give 100–200 mg at night, the effect lasting six to eight hours, and limit to a week or so.

Side-effects and interactions

Be cautious if renal or liver disease is present since these two organs normally terminate barbiturate action. Barbiturates are respiratory depressants and unsuitable in chronic bronchitis. Do not give to the elderly patient because of the risk of inducing disorientation.

Alcohol potentiates their effect and the two should never be taken together. The rare disease porphyria is exacerbated by them. Barbiturates stimulate liver enzymes and this leads to increased metabolism of other drugs. In the blood they may displace other drugs from their binding to plasma albumin.

The prescribing of barbiturates, as outlined above, is exceptional: always remember the risks of drug dependence, of death from accidental poisoning, especially in the elderly, the ill and the alcoholic, and where there is a risk of suicide.

Preparations

Tablets: 60 mg, 200 mg
Capsules: 60 mg, 200 mg
Injection: 250 mg and 500 mg powder in ampoules (for reconstitution).

Related drugs

Butobarbitone (Soneryl) (100 mg) is a hypnotic. Preparations containing quinal barbitone (Seconal and Tuinal) are now Schedule 2 drugs (Misuse of Drugs Regulations 1985). All prescribing must meet the special regulations (see pp. 43, 121) for controlled drugs.

Phenobarbitone and primidone (Mysoline) are described under "Anti-epileptic drugs" (pp. 209–210).

28 Other sedatives and hypnotics

Paraldehyde

This remains a safe, rapidly acting hypnotic even in the presence of poor renal function, since it is excreted predominantly in the breath. It is a potent sedative for the excited. It can be used to suppress epileptic fits, and to prevent abstinence symptoms in alcohol withdrawal, but is also able to induce dependence. People dislike its smell and taste. A rectal infusion, given as a 10% enema in saline, avoids this but may cause local irritation. A similar reaction can occur when taken orally. If giving it by deep intramuscular injection, beware of using plastic syringes, which it dissolves, and of damage to the sciatic nerve; abscess formation is particularly a risk. Whichever method, the dose is 5–10 ml. Avoid if liver damage or lung disease is present. The drug interacts with disulfiram (Antabuse).

Preparations

Paraldehyde draught BPC: 4 ml in 50 ml.
Injection: 5 ml ampoule; 10 ml ampoule.

Chloral hydrate

Chloral hydrate (Noctec, Welldorm) is metabolised in the body to the chlorine-substituted alcohol, trichloroethanol. This is a safe hypnotic, with few side-effects, short-acting and without hangover, and is particularly suitable for the elderly and physically frail. Do not prescribe for personality disorder, in which dependency occurs, and generally only use short term but avoid its use if there is severe cardiac, renal or hepatic disease.

Taken in water the mixture (0.5–2 g for insomnia) can be unpleasant to swallow because of the taste, and can cause gastric irritation. Adding milk may help, but a capsule (Noctec) or tablet (Welldorm) is better tolerated.

Preparations

Tablets: chloral betaine: 707 mg = 414 mg chloral hydrate
Capsules: 500 mg
Chloral mixture BPC: 5 ml
Elixir: 143 mg/5 ml.

Chlormethiazole

Chlormethiazole (Heminevrin) is a sedative drug. Although derived from part of the thiamine molecule it has no vitamin-like effect. It is widely used to control delirium tremens and withdrawal symptoms of drug addiction. Give 1500 mg every six hours for two days then 1000 mg every six hours for a further three days and finally 500 mg six-hourly for four more days, after which the drug should be stopped. Chlormethiazole induces dependence and so alcoholics and drug addicts readily develop a further addiction.

For daytime sedation, 500 mg is given thrice daily. The drug is suited for sleeplessness in the elderly as there is little hangover (dose 500–1000 mg) but again should be given for short periods only where other hypnotics fail.

Side-effects

It is a safe drug to use with no serious side-effects and low toxicity in overdose. Addiction is the most serious problem and hence the drug should not be used for longer than about a week. Sneezing, nasal tingling or burning, and conjunctival irritation occur, but are unimportant medically. Alcoholics who continue to drink when taking chlormethiazole risk death.

Preparations

Capsules: 192 mg chlormethiazole base (≡5 ml syrup)
Syrup: 250 mg/5 ml chlormethiazole edisylate.

Meprobamate

Since the advent of benzodiazepines, this mildly sedative drug (Equanil) has been less widely used. A thrice-daily dose of 400–800 mg reduces anxiety but use only for short-term treatment.

Side-effects

Drowsiness and impaired concentration can be a problem and dependency a more serious one. If withdrawn suddenly, fits may occur.

Preparations

Tablets: 200 mg, 400 mg.

Buspirone

Buspirone (Buspar), a recently introduced sedative, is unrelated to the benzodiazepines or to any other existing psychotropic drug. Anxiety symptoms are suppressed in seven to ten days, with a dose of 5–10 mg thrice daily, and not rapidly as with benzodiazepines. Tolerance is said not to develop, nor problematic withdrawal symptoms. Benzodiazepines should be withdrawn before starting buspirone. It is not anticonvulsant. Further experience is needed to evaluate its use more fully.

Dizziness, gastrointestinal upsets and headaches can occur, especially initially. Insomnia can be a problem.

Preparations

Tablets: 5, 10 mg.

29 Beta-blockers

Propranolol

Propranolol (Inderal, Apsolol, Berkolol, Bedranol SR, Sloprolol) may be used for:

(a) bodily symptoms of anxiety
(b) tremor.

Propranolol blockades peripheral beta-adrenergic receptors and in this way may relieve rapid pulse, palpitations, sweating and tremor. Neurotic patients who are troubled mainly by the bodily symptoms of anxiety are therefore more likely to be helped by propranolol than are those with mental symptoms of anxiety. Somatic symptoms arising from both acute panic attacks and chronic anxiety states can be relieved. The usual treatment is 10 mg, 20 mg or even 40 mg three or four times daily by mouth, beginning with the lower dose. Even higher doses may be tolerated. The drug penetrates the brain and may be sedative in high doses, but this is still uncertain.

High doses of up to 1000 mg have been claimed helpful in treating schizophrenia, but this may be a drug interaction since propranolol interferes with the degradative metabolism of chlorpromazine, slowing the process.

Propranolol may be effective for tremor not caused by anxiety, including lithium-induced tremor.

The beta-adrenergic blockade caused by propranolol reduces the pulse rate, but the rate should not go below 55 per minute. Bradycardia can be reversed by 1–2 mg of atropine intravenously. Treatment with propranolol should be discontinued by gradual dose reduction and not abrupt withdrawal, to avoid rebound tachycardia.

Side-effects and contraindications

Propranolol causes few side-effects in the physically healthy person. Light-headedness, visual and tactile hallucinations, tinnitus, erythematous skin rash and purpura have been reported. Propranolol can precipitate heart failure. If there is a history of cardiac disease, a cardiologist's advice should be sought before prescribing propranolol for anxiety. The drug interferes with the recognition of hypoglycaemia in the diabetic by preventing sweating and tachycardia. It may cause insomnia and/or depressive symptoms.

Asthma and obstructive airways disease contraindicate its use because of the risk of acute bronchospasm.

Preparations

Tablets: 10 mg, 40 mg, 80 mg, 160 mg
Sustained-release capsules: 80 mg, 160 mg.

Other related drugs

Atenolol (Tenormin)

Tablets: 25 mg, 50 mg, 100 mg (maximum daily dose 100 mg)

Oxprenolol (Trasicor)

Tablets: 20 mg, 40 mg, 80 mg, 160 mg
(maximum daily dose 160 mg daily)
Sustained-release capsules: 160 mg.

30 Anti-epileptic drugs

'Anticonvulsants' is the term given to a diverse group of chemicals which can control fits. The mechanism of their anticonvulsant action, preventing the spread of abnormal excitation in the brain, is not known. They may stabilise neuronal excitability by blocking the exchange of ions across membranes or by altering neurotransmitter levels. Barbiturates, phenytoin and carbamazepine are thought to have an effect on membranes; benzodiazepines, valproate, barbiturates and carbamazepine are believed to act on GABA mechanisms.

Anticonvulsants are small molecules absorbed from the gut with ease. They differ from each other in their rates of renal excretion, hepatic metabolism and fat solubility, factors determining drug levels in blood and brain. Carbamazepine and sodium valproate for example are rapidly metabolised and should be taken several times a day to maintain a therapeutic blood level, although brain drug levels may not fluctuate as rapidly as serum levels. In contrast, phenytoin, phenobarbitone and primidone are slowly metabolised and can be taken in a single daily dose. Some days or even weeks are needed after a change of dose to reach a new equilibrium. This is a reason why improvement may be delayed over a week after increasing a dose.

Competitive inhibition can result in one drug causing a rise in the serum level of another, while enzyme induction can cause a decrease. Phenytoin, barbiturate and carbamazepine in particular have these properties.

Most anticonvulsant drugs circulate in the blood partly free and partly bound to plasma proteins, the ratio of free to bound drug being a constant. When only one drug is taken, measuring the total serum concentration will serve as an estimate of free drug, the pharmacologically active fraction, but when more than one drug is taken, binding points on the plasma protein may be competed for and one drug may displace another. Carbamazepine may displace phenytoin for instance. This results in a higher fraction of the total serum phenytoin being unbound and active, with the possibility of toxicity from a dose formerly safe.

Metabolic adjustments including enzyme changes may take weeks to reach a steady state so clinical changes must be judged over a lengthy period. Some drug-induced metabolic changes can result in new disease. A few anticonvulsants stimulate the production of liver enzymes which prevent the conversion of dietary vitamin D to the metabolically active chemical. A person with a poor vitamin intake and no sunshine may be tipped into vitamin deficiency by long-term phenytoin or phenobarbitone. Phenytoin may divert folate from its metabolic role, resulting in a macrocytic anaemia. Porphyria may be precipitated by phenobarbitone, carbamazepine or phenytoin. Blood dyscrasias occur occasionally with nearly all the anticonvulsants.

Grand mal and partial seizures are usually well controlled by barbiturates or phenytoin. Phenytoin is preferred because of phenobarbitone's side-effects of sedation, increased irritability and cognitive impairment. Nowadays, carbamazepine is probably best because it has fewer side-effects. Sodium valproate is also effective in primary generalised fits. Petit mal responds to ethosuximide or sodium valproate. Temporal lobe epilepsy is more difficult to control; a combination of two drugs may be unavoidable.

Aim to use one drug to control fits (Table 4). Add a second only when one drug by itself has failed after a systematic trial. The prescription of more than two drugs concurrently results in a high frequency of side-effects, drug interactions, poor compliance and muddle about which drug is causing what effect.

TABLE 4
Guidelines for choice of drugs in epilepsy

Seizure type	*First choice*	*Second choice*
Grand mal (primary, generalised)	Carbamazepine Phenytoin Sodium valproate	Phenobarbitone (Primidone)
Petit mal	Ethosuximide Sodium valproate	Clonazepam
Partial (focal) motor/sensory	Carbamazepine Phenytoin	Phenobarbitone (Primidone)
Temporal lobe (partial, complex)	Carbamazepine Phenytoin	Phenobarbitone (Primidone)
Myoclonic/atonic	Sodium valproate Clonazepam	Ethosuximide
Status epilepticus	Diazepam	Chlormethiazole (Paraldehyde)

Drugs in parentheses are recommended only after the others have been tried.

Carbamazepine

Carbamazepine (Tegretol) may be used for:

(a) all forms of epilepsy except petit mal
(b) mood disturbance (see p. 150)
(c) trigeminal neuralgia.

For adults, give 200 mg daily, increasing the dose by 200 mg every two or three days depending on response. For most people 800–1200 mg is adequate, but a few may require 1600 mg a day. For children the dose ranges between 100 mg for infants to 1000 mg for 15-year-olds. Aim for a plasma level of 4–12 mg/l. Carbamazepine induces its own catabolic enzymes so serum levels may decline after a time on a constant dose, with the possibility of fits recurring. Carbamazepine should be avoided with atrioventricular conduction disorders and porphyrias.

Side-effects and interactions

Side-effects include gastrointestinal disturbances, nausea, headache, dizziness, drowsiness, ataxia, nystagmus, diplopia, and fluid retention. Leucopenia and blood dyscrasias have occurred. An itchy erythematous rash develops in about 5% but often disappears without stopping carbamazepine.

The drug is related to imipramine and may improve mood. Because of this similarity, in theory it should not be given with a monoamine oxidase inhibitor. Carbamazepine induces liver enzymes thereby reducing levels of clonazepam, ethosuximide and sodium valproate if taken concurrently with them. In the same way carbamazepine lessens the effectiveness of other drugs, including psychotropic drugs and itself. The dose of oral contraceptives and of warfarin may need raising. Some drugs, for example cimetidine, increase the metabolism of carbamazepine so reducing the serum level.

Preparations

Tablets: 100 mg, 200 mg, 400 mg
Slow-release tablets: 200 mg, 400 mg
Liquid: 100 mg/5 ml.

Phenytoin

Phenytoin (Epanutin) may be used for all types of epilepsy except petit mal.

For adults, and children over six years, 100 mg daily in one or two doses may be increased gradually to 600 mg daily depending on response. For children under six years, 5–8 mg/kg daily in one or two doses is recommended.

Several days are required to reach a stable level after each dose increase because of the long half-life. Phenytoin has a narrow therapeutic index. A small increase in dose may produce a large and toxic increase in serum level, and increase of dose should be linked with plasma monitoring. Because of saturation of the liver enzymes, aim for plasma levels of 10–20 mg/l. Patients sensitive to their facial appearance, adolescents especially, may not tolerate the facial coarsening, gum hyperplasia, acne and hirsutism.

Side-effects and interactions

Gastric upsets are common. At higher doses nystagmus, diplopia, vertigo, ataxic gait, and other cerebellar signs may occur, as can an acute brain syndrome, sometimes accompanied by dystonia and choreo-athetosis. Hyperplasia of gums develops in 20% of those on chronic treatment. Hirsutism, peripheral neuritis, skin rash and rarely folate-deficiency anaemia may develop. The folate deficiency can be treated with folic acid, permitting continuation of phenytoin.

Avoid giving phenytoin during pregnancy; primidone is preferable. Carbamazepine levels are lowered by concurrent prescription of phenytoin. Phenobarbitone interaction is complex, so in combined treatment check both drug levels after the dose of one is changed. Avoid rapid withdrawal.

Preparations

Tablets: 50 mg, 100 mg
Capsules: 25 mg, 50 mg, 100 mg
Chewable tablets (paediatric): 50 mg
Suspension: 30 mg/5 ml
Injection: 50 mg/ml in 5 ml ampoule.

Sodium valproate

Sodium valproate (Epilim) may be used to treat all forms of epilepsy. For adults, give 200 mg three times a day, increasing by 200 mg every third day according to response. Control of fits usually appears at 800–1400 mg but severe cases may need up to 2500 mg daily. For children the dose range is 400–1200 mg and for infants under three years 20–30 mg/kg per day. Clinical response is the best guide to dose. There is no true therapeutic range. Serum levels are useful for identifying the poor complier and for deciding to change to another drug when fit control is not achieved with a serum level above 150 mg/l.

Side-effects and interactions

Drowsiness, nausea, vomiting, increase in appetite and weight gain may occur. Fatal cases of acute liver disease have been reported, usually in patients with severe epilepsy who were or had been taking other anticonvulsants in combination. If there is any history of liver disease, check liver function regularly; if liver disease is active, avoid altogether. Serum phenobarbitone levels are raised when valproate is given with primidone or phenobarbitone, intensifying sedation. Sedation is marked when benzodiazepines are combined with valproate.

Preparations

Tablets: 100 mg, 200 mg, 500 mg
Syrup and liquid: 200 mg/5 ml
Injection: 400 mg per vial to mix with 4 ml water in ampoule.

Phenobarbitone

All forms of epilepsy except petit mal may be treated with phenobarbitone (Luminal). Phenobarbitone has now been superseded by phenytoin and carbamazepine as the drug of first choice in grand mal and partial seizures. Where it is to be used the adult dose is 60–200 mg a day and for children 5–8 mg/kg body weight, given at night to avoid sedation.

Aim for a plasma level of 15–40 mg/l. The drug is slowly metabolised by liver hydroxylases and takes three weeks to reach a stable blood level. Withdrawal should be slow, with a dose reduction of 60 mg every four weeks.

Side-effects and interactions

The initial sedation lessens as tolerance develops. Occasionally dexamphetamine is given to lessen sedation. Nystagmus, ataxia, and confusion may develop with big doses, especially in the elderly. Adults may show personality changes and children become irritable and overactive.

Oversedation may occur in the elderly and infirm. Breast-fed babies can become sleepy. It is unsuitable for alcoholics and those with impaired liver function. Phenobarbitone may reduce levels of other drugs (oestrogens, warfarin, valproate, tricyclics) by inducing extra production of liver hydroxylase. However, it may decrease the inactivation of phenytoin and raise its serum level.

Preparations

Tablets: 15 mg, 30 mg, 60 mg, 100 mg
Elixir: 15 mg/5 ml
Injection (phenobarbitone sodium): 200 mg/1 ml ampoule.

Primidone

Primidone (Mysoline) is converted to phenobarbitone in the liver, and this is why it is an anticonvulsant. Therefore do not combine it with phenobarbitone in treatment: note that all its side-effects are the same but more pronounced. It can be used for all forms of epilepsy except petit mal. Start with low doses, given at night to minimise side-effects, for adults use 125 mg increasing every third day by 125 mg to a level of 500–1500 mg daily, and for children allow 5–20 mg/kg.

Preparations

Tablets: 250 mg
Oral suspension: 250 mg/5 ml.

Ethosuximide

Ethosuximide (Zarontin, Emeside) is restricted to the treatment of petit mal. For adults start with 500 mg daily, increasing by 500 mg each week to 2000 mg according to response. In children under six years begin with 250 mg daily increasing to 1000 mg. Aim for a plasma level of 40–120 mg/l. Complete suppression of fits occurs in 50% of cases and partial suppression in 25%. If other types of fit coexist combine with carbamazepine, phenytoin or primidone.

Side-effects and interactions

Nausea, anorexia, headache, apathy, dizziness, sleepiness, mood changes, which are usually mild and diminish, skin rashes, and blood disorders may all occur.

Carbamazepine decreases plasma concentrations of ethosuximide and sodium valproate increases them.

Preparations

Capsules: 250 mg
Syrup: 250 mg/5 ml.

Clonazepam

Clonazepam (Rivotril) may be used for all forms of epilepsy. It is a benzodiazepine with a long half-life. For adults, start with 0.5 mg daily increasing by 0.5 mg every three days to a daily dose of 4–8 mg, depending on response. For children aged 5–12 years, use 3–6 mg daily, for children aged 1–5 years, 1–3 mg daily.

For status epilepticus, 1 mg by slow injection in an adult, 0.5 mg in a child is appropriate.

Side-effects and interactions

Drowsiness, which may be marked, can be lessened by giving at night and increasing the dose gradually. Giddiness, irritability, aggressiveness and diplopia are common.

Carbamazepine, phenobarbitone and phenytoin increase metabolism of clonazepam and serum levels of clonazepam are lowered. Avoid rapid withdrawal, which can precipitate status epilepticus.

Preparations

Tablets: 0.5 mg, 2 mg
Injection: 1 mg/1 ml ampoule.

Diazepam

Diazepam (Valium, Diazemuls, Stesolid) is best reserved for status epilepticus. By intravenous infusion as a 0.5% solution at a rate of 2.5 mg (0.5 ml) each 30 seconds, a dose of 10–20 mg should be administered depending on response. This may be repeated after 30–60 minutes. By rectum in solution, for adults and children over three years, the dose is 10 mg. For children under three years, 5 mg is appropriate, repeated if necessary.

Side-effects

Mechanical ventilation may be required when diazepam is given intravenously because of respiratory depression. (If diazepam or clonazepam is ineffectual in treating status epilepticus, i.v. chlormethiazole may be tried or paraldehyde given i.m. or rectally (see pp. 107, 198).)

Preparations

Injection: 5 mg/ml in 2 ml ampoule
Injection (emulsion): 5 mg/ml in 2 ml ampoule (Diazemuls)
Enema: 2 mg/ml and 4 mg/ml in 2.5ml rectal tubes (Stesolid).

Vigabatrin

Vigabatrin (Sabril) is recommended as an anticonvulsant for trial where other anti-epileptic drugs have failed. It is thought to act by raising GABA in the central nervous system by inhibiting GABA transaminase. Give 1.5–3 g per day.

Side-effects

Dizziness, unsteadiness, drowsiness may occur.

Preparations

Tablets: 500 mg.

31 Control of substance abuse

Disulfiram

Disulfiram (Antabuse) in combination with alcohol produces head throbbing, palpitations, tachycardia, facial flush, nausea, vomiting and sometimes dyspnoea. This very unpleasant experience, due to accumulation of acetaldehyde, is the basis of its use to discourage drinking in the alcoholic. Because of the potential severity of the reaction disulfiram is ideally restricted to the medically fit.

Disulfiram can be started with a challenge with alcohol under medical supervision, although in present practice the challenge tends to be dispensed with, and disulfiram (200 mg) is taken each morning as an out-patient, the patient being informed of the reaction to expect when alcohol is drunk. If the reaction with alcohol is absent or modest when the patient has a drink the dose can be increased to 400 mg. Success depends on a motivated, compliant patient using disulfiram as one, but not the sole aid, to control. Compliance is improved by enlisting a family member to help.

The alternative approach, using a challenge, relies to some extent for its effectiveness on a strong aversive experience. For the first three nights, 1.0 g disulfiram is taken, and thereafter 400 mg each morning. On the fifth morning, one hour after the last dose, give 15 ml of 95% alcohol diluted with the patient's favourite alcoholic drink. Within two hours the unpleasant experience should occur. The aim is to make a deep impression. If there is no adverse reaction, the dose can be increased and the challenge repeated. After the successful challenge, continue 400 mg disulfiram daily for three weeks, and then reduce to 200 mg daily indefinitely. The anti-alcohol effect lasts two days or more after the last dose of disulfiram. Severe reaction may be ended with 1g ascorbic acid orally or intravenously.

Side-effects and interactions

Without intake of alcohol, disulfiram may still produce drowsiness, fatigue, constipation, nausea, a garlic or metallic taste, smelly breath, and loss of libido. A smaller dose may reduce side-effects. The drug can also cause depressive hallucinatory or confusional symptoms. A severe alcohol reaction produces falling blood pressure, cardiac arrhythmias and collapse, and can be fatal. The small amounts of alcohol sometimes in oral medicines may produce a reaction. A patient's card, similar to that for monoamine oxidase inhibitors (MAOIs) (p. 155), may be useful.

Disulfiram interferes with the metabolism of other drugs, notably barbiturates, phenytoin and coumarin derivatives, increasing their pharmacological actions. Paraldehyde metabolism is blocked by disulfiram, yielding acetaldehyde, which produces a severe reaction.

Preparations

Tablets: 200 mg.

Methadone

Methadone (Physeptone), a synthetic opiate used in general medicine in placc of morphine for relieving pain and cough, is employed in psychiatry to manage opiate addiction. Although chemically distinct from other opiates, methadone has similar pharmacological properties which enable it to be substituted for heroin, etc. Controlled withdrawal is then easier to achieve using an oral drug with less severe withdrawal symptoms than the other opiates. The evidence for its value is based on uncontrolled trial and much clinical experience.

In divided doses, 40 mg per day is usually adequate to begin with: then attempt to reduce by 5 mg per day. The prescription must comply with the Controlled Drugs Regulations. Methadone is addictive and so can lead to lengthy if not indefinite maintenance. It may be deemed preferable to street opiates but this prescribing will depend on the policy of the local drug clinic (see p. 115).

Side-effects and interactions

Methadone, with a longer period of action than morphine, has similar side-effects but is not as sedative.

Methadone potentiates the sedative effects of alcohol, antidepressants, neuroleptics and other psychotropic drugs. Liver disease, renal disease, asthma and MAOI drugs are contraindications unless the reasons for long-term use are compelling. Hypertensive crises may occur with MAOI drugs.

Preparations

Tablets: 5 mg
Mixture: 1 mg/ml
Injection: 10 mg/ml.

Clonidine

Clonidine (Catapres, Dixarit), a central acting alpha-2-adrenergic agonist used to treat hypertension and migraine, is a useful adjunct in opiate withdrawal, suppressing autonomic symptoms without producing euphoria. Practice varies widely in its use both in withdrawal in acute phase and in longer-term management. Methadone can be prescribed simultaneously. Dosage is 100–600 μg daily.

Side-effects and interactions

Side-effects include drowsiness, dry mouth, oedema, bradycardia, and depression. Lactation may be inhibited. Peripheral vascular diseases may be worsened, for example in Raynaud's disease. Hypertensive crises may occur on rapid withdrawal.

Tricyclic antidepressants lessen its hypotensive effect.

Preparations

Tablets: 100 μg, 300μg
Sustained-release capsules: 250 μg
Injection: 150 μg/ml.

Naltrexone

Naltrexone (Nalorex), a centrally acting opiate-receptor blocker, has the clinically important property of preventing the 'buzz' experienced after taking an opiate. The principal reason for taking opiates illicitly, and which helps former addicts to become re-addicted, is therefore removed. Thus, naltrexone is beginning to find a place in the management of well motivated and co-operative patients who have been detoxified. The drug treatment forms one part of a co-ordinated team approach. Give 25–50 mg daily at first, under supervision, and then 100–150 mg on alternate days or every third day.

Side-effects and interactions

Nausea and vomiting, headache and sleeplessness may occur. Check hepatic function before and during treatment, and do not give the drug if there is any impairment. Patients should carry a drug warning card in case they need opiates for genuine pain relief.

Preparations

Tablets: 50 mg.

32 Anti-androgens

Cyproterone

Cyproterone acetate (Androcur), a powerful anti-androgen, competitively blocks androgens at receptor sites, including those in the brain. The blocking causes a reduction in circulating testosterone levels and reduced gonadotrophin levels. The reason for using the drug to control hypersexuality and deviant behaviour in the male is the assumption that such behaviour depends on androgen levels. The extent and nature of such a link in man is still unknown, but clinical experience suggests the drug can be useful in helping the well motivated male patient to control deviant sexual behaviour.

Cyproterone may have an effect on paedophilia, exhibitionism, fetishism, other deviant behaviour, and excessive demand for sexual intercourse if these practices are related to high sexual drive. Because of this, younger men are more likely to respond than older men. A dose of 100 mg daily (range 50–200 mg) is recommended, but assess patients every few days after each dose change. Drug treatment should be combined with psychological treatment directed to encouraging motivation to change and altering sexual preoccupations.

The use of cyproterone acetate raises ethical problems because of its intended effect to control an important part of behaviour. Only consenting patients should be treated, even in the case of a judicial treatment order. For detained patients, approval must be obtained from the Mental Health Act Commission (Maid Marian House,

56 Houndsgate, Nottingham NG1 1BR, tel. 0602-504 040), as required by the Mental Health Act 1983.

Side-effects and interactions

Tiredness is the main unwanted side-effect and is transient, but gynaecomastia, which may be irreversible, occurs in 20% of those given the drug. Reversible infertility is common, with increased numbers of abnormal spermatozoa. Whether abnormal offspring are born to fathers taking cyproterone is unknown, but the patient should be warned.

Cyproterone may cause liver damage and so should not be used for patients with liver disease, and liver function should be checked.

Preparations

Tablets: 50 mg.

Benperidol

Benperidol (Anquil) can be used in place of haloperidol in disturbed psychotic states, especially when associated with disinhibition and hypersexuality. It is also used in personality disorders with sexual deviation or abnormal sexual preoccupations but its effectiveness has not yet been established. Side-effects are as for butyrophenones (see p. 178) and dosage varies from 0.25 mg to 1.5 mg daily in divided doses.

Preparations

Tablets: 0.25 mg.

33 Vitamins

Prescribing vitamins for psychiatric patients is justified only when a vitamin deficiency state exists or there is strong suspicion that it does so. Vitamin deficiency states are uncommon in psychiatric patients, but a diet of poor quality or quantity, over a lengthy period, can lead to deficiency in the B group, vitamin C, vitamin B12 and folic acid.

Such a state results from the unsupervised self-neglect that occurs with dementia, the elderly mentally ill, chronic schizophrenia, and long-standing alcoholism, or from the deliberate self-starvation of anorexia nervosa and the extreme dietary practices resulting from delusional beliefs. An adequate diet, if the patient will have it, and vitamin supplements are all that are required to manage the deficiency, in the short term. A multiple vitamin preparation containing ascorbic acid, nicotinamide, pyridoxine, riboflavine and thiamine is often used. Folic acid may have to be prescribed if anaemia is present and this needs to be confirmed by a low red-cell folate level. Plasma folate levels indicate only current intake, not past deficiency. Dietary stores of vitamin B12 are usually large enough to withstand several years of poor diet.

Excessive intake of a vitamin may result from a delusion and be harmful and occasionally life-threatening, for example excessive amounts of carrot juice causing vitamin A poisoning.

Some psychiatric conditions result from vitamin deficiencies, although this is rare in Britain. Alcoholism and a poor diet may cause a thiamine deficiency which, if not urgently treated, damages mid-brain structures resulting in the Wernicke–Korsakov syndrome. Thiamine, given with other vitamins, prevents the syndrome from developing and probably shortens the delirium. Treatment is an urgent matter.

Pellagra, with its psychosis and dementia, is a rare consequence of nicotinamide deficiency. Dementia and cognitive impairment associated with deficiency of vitamin B12 or folic acid deficiency may respond partially to replacement therapy. The vitamin deficiency may not be causal but result from a poor diet brought about by a dementia. Pyridoxine is prescribed as a supplement to tryptophan when used as an antidepressant (but see p. 69) and also for pre-menstrual tension, but in neither case has its value been proved.

Many oral vitamin preparations are available. An injectable form, Parentrovite, is described here.

'Parentrovite'

'Parentrovite' may be used for

(a) delirium tremens
(b) Korsakov's psychosis and Wernicke's encephalopathy
(c) dietary deficiency states.

It is a proprietary preparation of thiamine (B1), riboflavine (B2), pyridoxine (B6), nicotinamide, and ascorbic acid (C) for parenteral use when vitamins are urgently required. For delirium tremens give pairs of intramuscular high-potency ampoules daily for five to seven days. Wernicke's encephalopathy as a medical emergency requires a more vigorous approach, with two to four pairs of ampoules being given intravenously every four to eight hours for up to 48 hours, depending on clinical response, followed by one pair of intravenous or intramuscular ampoules a day for five to seven days. For the less serious case and Korsakov's psychosis, a pair of intramuscular high-potency ampoules once or twice daily for up to seven days is sufficient until oral vitamin treatment can be given. Use only intravenous preparations for intravenous use and intramuscular preparations for intramuscular use.

Side-effects and interactions

Parentrovite is safe to use. Facial flushing occasionally results. Very large amounts may cause mental excitement which subsides when treatment stops. Anaphylaxis has been reported. Pyridoxine may destabilise the L-dopa treatment of Parkinson's disease.

Preparations

Intravenous, high potency

Ampoule 1, 5 ml: thiamine 250 mg, riboflavine 4 mg, pyridoxine 50 mg
Ampoule 2, 5 ml: nicotinamide 160 mg, ascorbic acid 500 mg, dextrose monohydrate 1000 mg.

Intramuscular, high potency

Vitamin composition as for intravenous high potency, but without dextrose, and with 140 mg benzyl alcohol, in two ampoules of 3.5 ml.

Intramuscular, maintenance

Ampoule 1, 2 ml: thiamine 100 mg, riboflavine 4 mg, pyridoxine 50 mg, benzyl alcohol 80 mg
Ampoule 2, 2 ml: nicotinamide 160 mg, ascorbic acid 500 mg.

Appendix 1. Consent to treatment

In general, all patients have the right to have a proposed treatment explained to them and to decide whether to accept it or not. However, psychiatric patients can pose two kinds of difficulty here.

(a) Some psychiatric patients may consent although they have not understood the explanation or what they are agreeing to. Perhaps they agree to please the doctor, or are giving way to what they feel is pressure, or they regard the treatment as a punishment which they believe they fully deserve. This is not real consent; it is termed 'incompetent' and is not acceptable.

(b) Others fail to give consent not because they necessarily disagree but because the very nature of their illness makes it impossible. They may be mute, or in catatonic stupor, or suffer from a state of continuous indecision about everything, or entertain bodily delusions, or have a marked thought disorder which makes it very difficult to be sure what they mean when they speak.

Yet it may truly be in the patient's best interests to have the proposed treatment, or it may even be a matter of death if they do not have it.

With incompetent consent, or none, treatment would be an assault and illegal. The Mental Health Act 1983 (MHA) provides a way out, a procedure allowing treatment of the non-consenting patient by making safeguards for both patient and medical and nursing staff. The patient must be detained under a section of the Act (which means they must show certain abnormalities recognised by two separate doctors), and the treatment must be approved by an independent consultant from the Mental Health Act Commission (MHAC). An informal patient in hospital may have to be detained for this purpose, and this will need the opinions of a doctor approved under Section 12 of the Act as having special knowledge of psychiatry, and of another doctor who is not on the hospital staff, most often the family doctor. Section 2 of the MHA lasts 28 days, and Section 3 lasts six months; both can be cancelled at any time before they expire. Mentally abnormal offenders detained through a court under sections 36, 37, 38, 47, or 48 also satisfy the legal requirements.

The patient is then assessed by the independent consultant appointed by the MHAC, and approval for treatment is given or not.

This procedure, with second opinions, can take time, especially at weekends. In dire emergency the common law allows doctors to act for the patient on their own initiative alone, avoiding the Act's procedure. For instance, a very depressed and seriously dehydrated patient refusing all fluids could justifiably receive electroconvulsive therapy (ECT) forthwith to get drinking started again. Where a patient is already detained, Section 62 of the Act allows ECT to be given without MHAC prior approval in an emergency, for instance where the risk of suicide is very high. In practice, this usually means the first ECT only is given as, by the second, a MHAC consultant will have assessed the patient. The keeping of full written records of what is being done at all times is an important additional safeguard. The patient's relatives should also be kept fully informed; it is hoped they will concur in the treatment, but their approval is not needed, and they cannot bar it.

The treatments controlled by the Act and discussed here are: ECT, psychotropic drug injections, and the surgical implant of sex hormones to reduce male sex drive. Leucotomy, a purely surgical procedure, is also controlled but is outside the scope of this book. The procedures outlined apply to England and Wales; similar practices are followed in other parts of the UK.

Electroconvulsive therapy

It is the responsibility of the doctor (not a nurse) to explain to the patient and relative why the treatment is necessary, how it is given, and the effects expected. This should be done in all cases, even where there is doubt over whether the patient can understand, or is refusing. The doctor signs a form to say he/she has explained, and the patient signs, or refuses to, in which case this is noted. A record should also be made about the assessment of the patient's competence. When a detained patient gives consent, a special form is signed by the consultant stating the patient is in a fit state to make a decision and has agreed.

If the patient consents, it permits a series of eight to ten treatments. Fresh consent will be needed for any further series and particularly if treatment is to be resumed after a gap of at least 21 days. The patient may at any time withdraw consent, and treatment then stops.

If the patient is uncertain about consenting, respect this uncertainty and leave the matter a while. Try again later: when they see they are not to be forced, and appreciate that ECT may be their only road to recovery or at least to getting out of hospital, they may agree after all.

If the patient is incompetent to consent, or refuses to agree, and ECT is clearly needed, he/she must be detained, if not already so, and approval for ECT sought from the MHAC consultant (Section 53(3)(b)). The case should also be discussed with the ECT team (anaesthetist and nurses) so that they know how important the treatment is, and how far to go with a seemingly unwilling patient. Most patients will go along with treatment once all the paperwork has been done. It is a mistake to fight in the ECT room with a patient still determined to refuse. This should not arise if matters have been explained in a friendly way all along, particularly if a known nurse or doctor accompanies the patient to the ECT room and can talk with the patient encouragingly. Occasionally sedation before treatment (e.g. 2 mg oral diazepam) may be helpful.

More detailed and useful information is given by the ECT Sub-committee of the Research Committee, Royal College of Psychiatrists (1989).

Drug injections

Drugs may be injected without consent if the patient is detained. After three months' treatment so begun, the responsible medical officer must sign a certificate that the patient understands the nature, purpose and effects of the drug and agrees to continue. Otherwise a second opinion must be obtained from a MHAC consultant (Sections 58(1)b and (3)b). Long-stay in-patients may agree to treatment without understanding, so it is wise to have a written second opinion if there is the slightest doubt.

Out-patients

Patients discharged on successful treatment with depot injections usually willingly continue with them thereafter if only because of a good relationship with the staff and/or as part of some continuing social treatment programme. A few do not however, and they may relapse and have to be readmitted. It is not legal to try to prevent relapse using drugs with a non-consenting patient. They can have no further treatment against their wishes unless, on assessment, their symptoms are of such severity to warrant action under Section 2 or 3 of the MHA. A Guardianship Order (Sections 7 and 8) can require a patient to attend for treatment but does not authorise any treatment, including drugs, against the patient's wishes. A probation order with a condition of treatment imposed by a court likewise does not compel the acceptance of medication.

Implant of hormones

Surgical implant of hormones (but not of drugs) to reduce sex drive requires for all patients, whether detained or not, the patient's agreement plus a MHAC consultant's approval (Section 57).

Reference

ECT Sub-Committee of the Research Committee (1989) *The Practical Administration of Electroconvulsive Therapy (ECT)*. London: Royal College of Psychiatrists.

Appendix 2. Electroconvulsive therapy, continuous sleep and abreaction

How to give electroconvulsive therapy

A series of induced epileptic fits, spaced at two- or three-day intervals, is an effective treatment for serious depressive illness. Given more frequently electroconvulsive therapy (ECT) suppresses mania, and one or two fits are enough to abolish catatonic stupor or an acute brain syndrome. Combined with a phenothiazine it can be more effective in schizophrenia than phenothiazine by itself. Why fits are therapeutic is unknown. It is simply an observed fact of human biology.

It is the fit and not the electricity of ECT that is the agent, because fits from an intravenous drug like Metrazol or an inhaled vapour – hexafluorodiethyl ether or Indoklon – are also therapeutic. Stimulation of a fit by brief pulses of current to the head is least unpleasant to the patient and most easily controlled, but there is evidence that the size of the pulse (the electric charge) may matter too, whereas duration of fit probably does not. The tonic and clonic muscle contractions of a convulsion are unnecessary (and if violent may result in fractures), so they are suppressed by giving a small dose of a muscle relaxant or paralyser acting at the motor end-plates.

Commonly succinyl choline is used; it is normally quickly destroyed by a pseudocholine esterase in the blood, so its action is brief. It is usually given under cover of anaesthesia with a short-acting intravenous barbiturate (thiopentone or methohexitone).

For therapeutic effect the fit must be bilateral and major in type, but what matters is the epileptic disturbance in the brain. Twitching of both thumbs and both big toes is simply an indicator to the operator that a major fit is occurring. A useful technique is to apply a sphygmomanometer cuff to one arm (same side as unilateral electrodes) and block blood flow (above systolic blood pressure). This is done before giving the intravenous drugs, so that muscles distal to the cuff cannot receive relaxant. They can thus contract rhythmically when the epileptic discharge begins, even though the fit would be otherwise invisible because of the complete paralysis of the rest of the body muscles produced by the relaxant.

The treatment is physically safe, can be given to: the very old, the frail, the pregnant, and those with hypertension, cardiac arrythmia, cardiac failure, Parkinson's disease, and previous stroke or myocardial infarction (the last two 12 weeks or more after the attack). Since ECT with relaxant still produces brief rises in blood pressure, treatment of patients with aneurysms, recent cerebral haemorrhage or raised intracranial pressure should be regarded with very great caution, and avoided if possible.

The patient should be assessed the day after each treatment, and treatment concluded when no further benefit appears. In depressive illness there may be no change until after the first two or three treatments, when some improvement suddenly appears, and six or eight in all may be enough. Never give fixed courses. Patients differ. The elderly and brain-damaged are more likely to suffer memory disturbance. Too much ECT may result in hypomania, an acute brain syndrome, or restless anxiety. Fortunately these usually clear in seven to ten days and without additional medication. In schizophrenia a longer series of treatments, perhaps up to 12, may sometimes be needed.

Procedure

Explain the treatment to patient and relative, and get the necessary forms signed as evidence of consent. See Appendix 1 on consent to treatment.

Discuss with the ECT team beforehand if there are any problems about consent and with the anaesthetist about any medical condition of the patient and about drugs already being taken (especially monoamine oxidase inhibitors, which affect resuscitative measures).

Check the patient's dental state. False teeth should be removed before treatment, but decayed teeth may break in a fit and a piece be inhaled, so dental care beforehand may be indicated.

As before any general anaesthetic, the patient fasts overnight, but may have a cup of tea three hours beforehand. Diabetics require special arrangements: they will continue with regular insulin and glucose and have their ECT by convenient timed appointment.

The hair must be free from grease and lacquer and the skin clean, to make good electrical contact with the electrodes. All metal objects (hair grips, glasses) must be removed to avoid short-circuits.

If the patient has a cold or respiratory infection on the morning of treatment, treatment must be postponed for another day. A nervous or doubtful patient may be encouraged by the presence and supportive conversation of a nurse or doctor he/she knows. Sometimes a small dose of a benzodiazepine an hour beforehand may be helpful, but possibly may raise seizure threshold.

The treatment is given to each patient, singly, in a separate room with the door closed. The sight or the sound of a person receiving ECT and the comments of the ECT team can alarm those waiting. Separate waiting, treatment and recovery rooms are ideal.

Before the patient comes into the treatment room, make yourself familiar with the ECT machine and its calibration. Examine the patient's ECT form, which ought to show information relevant to giving anaesthetic and ECT, in particular drug treatment and medical conditions. The notes of previous ECT will show:

(a) the doses of muscle relaxant and anaesthetic found effective
(b) the setting on the ECT machine that gave a fit
(c) the non-dominant side if the patient is to have unilateral ECT
(d) problems such as difficulty in finding a vein, failure to get a fit, prolonged apnoea.

Fresh entries are made after each treatment.

The patient receives, from the anaesthetist, the anaesthetic and relaxant and, when unconscious, a few squeezes of oxygen from the re-breathing bag. A gag is then placed between the teeth to protect the tongue. The relaxant causes muscles to fasciculate. Wait a few moments for this to die away.

The electrodes are then applied to the head, either one on each side (bilateral) or both on the same side (unilateral), the non-dominant side of the cerebrum (Fig. 9). The first is technically a little easier and slightly more effective, the second has the advantage of quicker recovery after the fit and far less risk of memory disturbance. But which is the non-dominant side? In right-handed people, and in two-thirds of left-handed

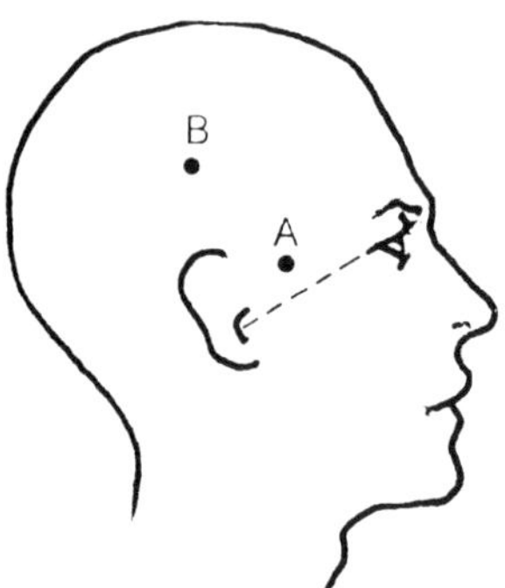

Fig. 9. Unilateral ECT: electrodes are placed (A) 4 cm above midpoint between earhole and angle of eye, and (B) 6 cm from A, above ear

or ambidextrous people, it is the right-hand side of the head; in the rest it is the left-hand side. Asking about or testing for hand, foot and eye preference usually shows dominance. Otherwise, give the first unilateral treatment to the left side and the second to the right side, and compare the after-effects; continue treatments on the side with less disturbance. The electrodes must be well moistened to conduct evenly, otherwise the current may not pass or may cause a skin burn. On the other hand, if they are very wet, fluid will run on the skin and may allow a short circuit. Press them firmly into the cleansed skin with a slight twist and hold them there until the fit is over. (Recent work suggests that electrodes bifrontally, i.e. 5 cm above external angle of orbit on each side, produces fits more effectively than when applied unilaterally, but with a similar lack of memory disturbance.)

Press the ECT button. The immediate muscle twitch is a direct response to the current and not a fit, but after about 10 seconds, or longer, a rhythmic jerking begins in the eyelids, thumbs and toes. It dies away after about 40 seconds and the patient lies relaxed and apnoeic. Movement must be bilaterally symmetrical even with unilateral stimulation to be a sign of an effective fit.

If no fit has occurred, repeat the stimulation once at a much higher electrical setting. If this fails, postpone a fresh try to another day. Each electric shock adds to the side-effects.

Thresholds for fits vary. Fit threshold is raised by drugs with anticonvulsant properties, such as benzodiazepines, dehydration, previous ECT, and old age. Dry electrodes, dirty skin, or oily hair can insulate from the electric shock and cause fit failure with an apparently satisfactory setting.

When the fit is over, oxygen is given after inserting an airway. Shortly afterwards the patient begins to breathe. After the resumption of spontaneous breathing the patient is turned on one side and transferred to a recovery room for post-anaesthetic care. A nurse must be present until consciousness returns and post-fit confusion settled enough for the patient to be safe alone.

Recovery of spontaneous breathing is sometimes delayed. Artificial respiration will then have to be continued. Delayed recovery beyond 30 minutes is an anaesthetic emergency requiring intubation and transfer to intensive care. Delay can result from too much muscle relaxant, rarely because of pseudocholinesterase deficiency. Recovery to consciousness takes a few minutes, the time depending on the anaesthetic drug and its dose, other sedative drugs, age, and state of health.

Brief confusion, restlessness, headache and nausea are common following ECT. A cup of tea, a lie-down, an aspirin may help these after-effects disappear. Assessment for therapeutic benefit should be made next day, after each treatment. Amnesia for events immediately before ECT and patchy losses of memory after ECT, most often for less important matters, is common. Memory difficulties usually subside in two or three weeks but may persist for longer. Depressive illness does itself appear to be associated with memory impairment and distinguishing between this and an ECT effect may be impossible.

Sometimes the anaesthetist cannot insert a needle into a vein. The insertion of an in-dwelling cannula for the duration of the course of ECT is a possible plan. Formerly, ECT might be given without anaesthesia or relaxant (unmodified ECT) if the patient became distressed by repeated failure to find a vein. This is no longer justifiable in general. Exceptionally, however, circumstances may arise when unmodified ECT should be used and we have included an account.

The psychiatrist must decide when to give the unmodified ECT. At a pre-agreed signal, nurses should gently but firmly hold the patient, leaning across hips and shoulders and holding the arms. Apply the electrodes and without delay give the shock. A typical grand mal convulsion results. Insert an airway when the convulsion has ceased, and give post-anaesthetic care. Because ECT produces amnesia for events just before the shock patients will not recall what happened. Properly carried out unmodified ECT is not frightening to the patient, nor unpleasant. The increased risk of side-effects of the convulsion, however, have to be considered and weighed against the expected benefits.

Electroconvulsive therapy is a medical treatment given for serious mental illness. Ultimately the psychiatrist, after consulting with the anaesthetist, must balance the need for ECT against the risks of giving ECT and then decide whether to give it and under what circumstances.

Continuous sleep

The ancient notion of a period of rest as a medical treatment for agitation, anxiety or distress guided practice before contemporary treatments such as ECT and psychotropic drugs. Nowadays, prolonged sleep may still have a use in dealing with episodes of overwhelming anxiety following the stress of exposure to a disaster or experiencing bereavement. Sleep may also have a place in the treatment of severe obsession or overwhelming and frequent panic attacks. Depressive illness, mania, schizophrenia or organic states are most unlikely to benefit. The aim is sleep for 20 out of 24 hours for 3–20 days. The risks are bronchopneumonia, cardiovascular collapse, urinary retention, toxic overdosage. To minimise risks continuous sleep must be managed in a careful, disciplined way by skilled and experienced staff. Nursing should be in a quiet, dark, warm, single room. The sleep schedule is five hours' sleep followed by one awake repeated through the 24 hours. Each break has the same sequence, a gentle awakening, recording of pulse, temperature, blood pressure, getting out of bed for a walk, passing urine, and an opportunity to defaecate. On three out of the four awakenings a meal and on the fourth a glucose drink are given. Then more drugs are administered, the lights dimmed and the patient goes to sleep again. A fluid chart record must be kept systematically with the aim of a daily intake of 2.5 litres.

The drugs are a phenothiazine combined with a hypnotic, the exact choice a matter of experience, the dose judged according to the patient's response. Changes of dose are frequent, in the first day or so to find the dose that ensures sleep and then to the maintenance dose that avoids overdosage but continues sleep. Usually the drug doses can be gradually and considerably reduced from day to day as the patient achieves a pattern of sleeping.

A possible regime is 100 mg oral chlorpromazine and either 300 mg sodium amylbarbitone or 20 mg diazepam, every six hours for the first 48 hours. The supervising doctor, who must be experienced in this treatment, should see the patient three times in the 24 hours and always be available for consultation by nursing staff to assess complications.

During wakefulness some psychotherapy can be attempted, aimed at the resolution of social or emotional difficulties. The relationship which develops may assist future psychotherapy.

If the pulse increases, the blood pressure falls, temperature rises, other signs of physical illness develop, or the patient becomes delirious, the sedation should cease and the patient allowed to awaken.

Abreaction

A dose of anaesthetic insufficient to anaesthetise produces a state of altered consciousness, calm, relaxed, dreamy, inattentive to surroundings, and more suggestible. This state induces freer, less guarded speech and can be used as a diagnostic aid for mute states or as an adjunct to psychotherapy. The technique has been called 'narcoanalysis' or 'narcohypnosis', and 'abreaction' when accompanied by the display of strong emotion.

Mute states not due to neurological or medical causes are usually hysterical fugues or psychoses. An abreaction may enable the diagnosis, the forgotten identity being recalled or abnormal psychotic experiences and thinking being revealed. The discovery of delusions, abnormal thinking, or abnormal experiences thus allows appropriate treatment for a depressive illness or schizophrenia.

In fugue states the recollection of identity may be accompanied by remembrance of unpleasant events preceding the memory loss, with emotional display and subsequent improvement. Persons of previously good personality whose symptoms began following a distressing event, cases of post-traumatic neuroses for example, may re-experience the event. Emotions allowed open expression and re-enactment may lose their force and clinical improvement may result.

A barbiturate or benzodiazepine by intravenous injection is the safest and easiest drug to use. With sodium amylobarbitone, 250 mg in 5 ml or 500 mg in 10 ml is usually enough. The injection is given intravenously at the rate of 1 ml per minute while talking to the patient and noting respiration. Other drugs are 2.5% solution of sodium thiopentone, starting with 3 ml intravenously and then at the rate of 1 ml per minute up to 15 ml, or 10–20 mg diazepam intravenously over several minutes.

Talking may begin with suggestions of comfort and relaxation and asking about the effects of the injection; a heavy sigh is often the sign of the drug acting. Then proceed to ask about neutral matters of personal history before moving on to incidents or topics of emotional concern. Do not give more drug than necessary to reach the relaxed state or the patient may go into a long sleep and forget. If important memories are recalled, keep the patient talking until the drug effect wears off, so that the recollection is maintained in full consciousness. After recovery from the drug, discussion of the material uncovered helps to re-establish and re-integrate the forgotten material.

Appendix 3. People who take overdoses

Self-poisoning, admitted or discovered, raises the questions of future suicide (to be prevented) and of life stresses (to be alleviated). All people who take overdoses require assessment from these two points of view, whether or not they require revival. Revival is a medical matter, perhaps in accident and emergency or a medical ward, and comes first; psychiatric assessment should be carried out there or at least begun there. Bear in mind the following.

(a) Some patients claim the overdose was an accident, or taken only to get some sleep, and without lethal intent. It is dangerous to accept this at face value, and they should be assessed like all other overdosers.

(b) Unless the patient works with drugs, he/she is likely to have some mistaken ideas of what is dangerous, and the actual dose of drug taken is not a reliable guide to assess the degree of suicidal intent. Someone who takes only very few tablets may firmly intend death. Additionally, mental illness may mean indecision and sudden reversals of actions, resulting in incomplete dosing. All who have taken *anything* should be assessed.

(c) Overdosers have to be sorted into one of the following.

(i) Those who intended to die, but failed through accident, insufficient knowledge, or indecision. They may try again. They divide into: those with a prolonged intent, perhaps evident in long pre-planning; those with short, possibly recurrent periods of death intent; and those with extremely brief impulsive actions.

(ii) Those who were not thinking positively of death, but

wanting to escape from some seemingly hopeless situation, to let fate decide the future, or to test the attitudes of others.

(iii) A few who use suicidal threats and acts to gain enjoyable dramatic attention or to manipulate their relatives, doctors and others.

(iv) A few who attempt suicide as a social response in a particular cultural setting: a successful city man facing financial ruin or prosecution may try to kill himself.

(d) Group (i) carry the big risk of suicide, soon or later, and should have psychiatric care, probably ward admission. Group (iii) will repeat overdosing while the response is gratifying, a dangerous practice which could be lethal.

(e) The initial assessment is to decide the sort of person the patient is – whether impulsive, intelligent, a planner; whether subject to mental illness – looking for the presence of serious depressive illness (with biological symptoms such as insomnia, loss of appetite, inability to do usual work, loss of all feelings and delusions of illness or guilt), or of schizophrenia, or of alcoholism with its problems. A medical and psychiatric history (including family history) is needed, with any evidence of thoughtless impulsive personality or alcohol or drug abuse, and the present mental state.

(f) Much of this information should be obtained from relative or friend even before the patient recovers consciousness. It will include detail of when, where and how secretly the overdose was taken; and whether the patient showed any change from usual behaviour in the two days or more beforehand.

(g) At this stage some practitioners assess the environmental and emotional stresses the patient has recently been subject to, and sympathise for example with a dreadful marriage or catastrophic loss of job. While relevant to later assessment, this is dangerously mistaken because it leads to an underestimate of suicidal risk. 'Understanding' the basis for the patient's act can lead to empathy but confuse the issue of risk. What matters is not the stresses, if any, on the patient but purely what the patient's weakness is at present, as shown by the current symptoms in variety and duration. Weakness predicts risk, but so does determination.

(h) A small diagnostic problem arises with patients who have for long been chronic surgery attenders, with insomnia of some degree, anxiety, psychosomatic symptoms or hypochondriacal complaints. A more serious acute depression may have quietly emerged, but may not be recognised except by inquiring for new symptoms, including those of a biological nature. If not, the wrong assumption of a continued mild neuroticism will be made. Everlasting complainers unable to accept help but continuing to complain may turn to suicide when they see everyone is exhausted and no longer tolerant of them.

(i) The later assessment, exploration of the personal relationships, work, housing, and life of the patient generally to discover what stresses there are, is particularly necessary for groups (ii) and (iii) above. Social work may alter some of the stresses, supportive or educational psychotherapy help in their toleration. The act of the overdose itself may precipitate changes which satisfy the patient, and no further management is needed, but give time for relatives or friends to rally round; discharge from hospital before this can occur may lead to a repeated act.

(j) For those who remain a risk and are discharged home, clarify who is the key professional worker to provide continuity, e.g. community nurse, hospital doctor, general practitioner, social worker. Clear communication with them and with the patient's family is essential.

(k) Assessment of overdosers can be haphazard in general hospitals, perhaps not done at all, or by junior staff without psychiatric experience. One consultant psychiatrist should be responsible for setting up a service to provide systematic assessment of suicide in accident and emergency or medical wards. Assessment can be by nurses, social workers or junior doctors provided the consultant ensures that they receive the essential brief training.

(l) The Mental Health Act 1983 used to admit patients to hospital against their will is especially relevant to overdoses in category (i), above.

Appendix 4. Other sources of information

More detailed and invaluable up-to-date information on the clinical use and cost of drugs is contained in the *British National Formulary* (BNF), published by the British Medical Association and the Royal Pharmaceutical Society of Great Britain several times a year, and issued regularly to medical practitioners. It also provides the telephone numbers of drug information services and for the emergency treatment of poisoning. There is general guidance on prescribing and more specific details for prescribing controlled drugs. Regulations are altered from time to time and it is important to check the up-to-date rules by referring to the most recent BNF.

The *Monthly Index of Medical Specialities* (MIMS), published by Haymarket Publishing Ltd, London, also gives lists of drugs and their costs but with very limited information on clinical use.

Other references

AYD, F. J. & BLACKWELL, B. (1984) *Discoveries in Biological Medicine.* New York: Ayd Medical Community.

DUKES, M. N. G. (ed.) *Meyler's Side Effects of Drugs* (11th edn). Amsterdam: Excerpta Medica.

—— & BEALEY, L. (1989) *Side Effects of Drugs Annual* (11th edn, vols 1–13). Amsterdam: Elsevier.

GILMAN, A. G., *et al* (1985) *The Pharmacological Basis of Therapeutics* (7th edn). New York: Macmillan.

Index 1: Names of drugs

The proprietary or trade names are given in italics; the page numbers for the main entries are listed first.

Index 2: Symptoms and usages

The page numbers for the main entries are listed first. Only approved drug names are given. (ECT = electroconvulsive therapy; MAOI = monoamine oxidase inhibitors; LSD = lysergic acid diethylamide.)